Diabetes and Aging

Editor

ELSA S. STROTMEYER

CLINICS IN
GERIATRIC MEDICINE

www.geriatric.theclinics.com

February 2015 • Volume 31 • Number 1

ELSEVIER

1600 John F. Kennedy Boulevard • Suite 1800 • Philadelphia, Pennsylvania, 19103-2899

http://www.theclinics.com

CLINICS IN GERIATRIC MEDICINE Volume 31, Number 1
February 2015 ISSN 0749–0690, ISBN-13: 978-0-323-35439-4

Editor: Jessica McCool
Developmental Editor: Colleen Viola

Clinics in Geriatric Medicine (ISSN 0749-0690) is published quarterly by Elsevier Inc., 360 Park Avenue South, New York, NY 10010-1710. Months of issue are February, May, August, and November. Business and Editorial Offices: 1600 John F. Kennedy Blvd., Suite 1800, Philadelphia, PA 191023-2899. Periodicals postage paid at New York, NY, and additional mailing offices. Subscription prices are $280.00 per year (US individuals), $498.00 per year (US institutions), $145.00 per year (US student/resident), $370.00 per year (Canadian individuals), $632.00 per year (Canadian institutions), $195.00 per year (Canadian student/resident), $390.00 per year (international individuals), $632.00 per year (international institutions), and $195.00 per year (international student/resident). Foreign air speed delivery is included in all Clinics subscription prices. All prices are subject to change without notice. POSTMASTER: Send address changes to Clinics in Geriatric Medicine, Elsevier Health Sciences Division, Subscription Customer Service, 3251 Riverport Lane, Maryland Heights, MO 63043. Telephone: 1-800-654-2452 (U.S. and Canada); 314-447-8871 (outside U.S. and Canada). Fax: 314-447-8029. E-mail: journalscustomerservice-usa@elsevier. com (for print support) or journalsonlinesupport-usa@elsevier.com (for online support).

Reprints. For copies of 100 or more, of articles in this publication, please contact the Commercial Reprints Department, Elsevier Inc., 360 Park Avenue South, New York, New York 10010-1710. Tel.: 212-633-3874; Fax: 212-633-3820, E-mail: reprints@elsevier.com.

Clinics in Geriatric Medicine is covered in MEDLINE/PubMed (Index Medicus), EMBASE/Excerpta Medica, Current Contents/Clinical Medicine (CC/CM), and the Cumulative Index to Nursing & Allied Health Literature.

Contributors

EDITOR

ELSA S. STROTMEYER, PhD, MPH
Assistant Professor, Center for Aging and Population Health, Department of Epidemiology, Graduate School of Public Health, University of Pittsburgh, Pittsburgh, Pennsylvania

AUTHORS

R. NISHA AURORA, MD
Assistant Professor of Medicine, Division of Pulmonary, Critical Care, and Sleep Medicine, Johns Hopkins University, School of Medicine, Baltimore, Maryland

JOSHUA I. BARZILAY, MD
Professor, Kaiser Permanente, Duluth, Georgia; Division of Endocrinology, Emory University School of Medicine, Atlanta, Georgia

SHERI R. COLBERG, PhD
Human Movement Sciences Department, Old Dominion University, Norfolk, Virginia

NATHALIE DE REKENEIRE, MD, MS
Section of Geriatrics, Department of Internal Medicine, Yale School of Medicine, New Haven, Connecticut

KRISTA L. DONOHOE, PharmD, BCPS, CGP
Assistant Professor, Geriatrics, Department of Pharmacotherapy & Outcomes Science, Virginia Commonwealth University, Richmond, Virginia

G. KELLEY FITZGERALD, PhD, PT, FAPTA
Professor, Department of Physical Therapy, School of Health and Rehabilitation Sciences, University of Pittsburgh, Pittsburgh, Pennsylvania

JEFFREY B. HALTER, MD
Professor of Internal Medicine; Director, Division of Geriatric and Palliative Medicine, University of Michigan Geriatrics Center, Ann Arbor, Michigan

DEBORAH A. JOSBENO, PhD, PT, NCS
Assistant Professor, Department of Physical Therapy, School of Health and Rehabilitation Sciences, University of Pittsburgh, Pittsburgh, Pennsylvania

SAMANNAAZ S. KHOJA, PT, MS
PhD Candidate, Department of Physical Therapy, School of Health and Rehabilitation Sciences, University of Pittsburgh, Pittsburgh, Pennsylvania

JORGE R. KIZER, MD, MSc
Associate Professor, Departments of Medicine and Epidemiology and Population Health, Albert Einstein College of Medicine, Bronx, New York

ANNEMARIE KOSTER, PhD
Associate Professor, Department of Social Medicine, CAPHRI School for Public Health and Primary Care, Maastricht University, Maastricht, The Netherlands

ELIZABETH ROSE MAYEDA, PhD, MPH
Postdoctoral Fellow, Department of Epidemiology and Biostatistics, University of California, San Francisco, San Francisco, California

KAROLINE MOON, MD
Fellow, Division of Pulmonary, Critical Care, and Sleep Medicine, Johns Hopkins University, School of Medicine, Baltimore, Maryland

STEVEN MORRISON, PhD
School of Physical Therapy and Athletic Training, Old Dominion University, Norfolk, Virginia

KENNETH J. MUKAMAL, MD, MPH
Associate Professor, Department of Medicine, Beth Israel Deaconess Medical Center, Harvard University, Boston, Massachusetts

KELECHI C. OGBONNA, PharmD, CGP
Assistant Professor, Geriatrics, Department of Pharmacotherapy & Outcomes Science, Virginia Commonwealth University, Richmond, Virginia

MIJUNG PARK, PhD, MPH, RN
Assistant Professor, Department of Health and Community Systems, University of Pittsburgh School of Nursing, Pittsburgh, Pennsylvania

EMILY P. PERON, PharmD, MS, BCPS, FASCP
Assistant Professor, Geriatrics, Department of Pharmacotherapy & Outcomes Science, Virginia Commonwealth University, Richmond, Virginia

SARA R. PIVA, PhD, PT, OCS, FAAOMPT
Associate Professor, Department of Physical Therapy, School of Health and Rehabilitation Sciences, University of Pittsburgh, Pittsburgh, Pennsylvania

NARESH M. PUNJABI, MD, PhD
Professor of Medicine, Division of Pulmonary, Critical Care, and Sleep Medicine, Johns Hopkins University, School of Medicine, Baltimore, Maryland

CHARLES F. REYNOLDS III, MD
UPMC Endowed Professor of Geriatric Psychiatry, Department of Psychiatry, University of Pittsburgh School of Medicine; Director, NIMH Center of Excellence in Late Life Depression Prevention and Treatment, Hartford Center of Excellence in Geriatric Psychiatry, and Aging Institute of UPMC Senior Services and University of Pittsburgh, Pittsburgh, Pennsylvania

AMY E. ROTHBERG, MD, PhD
Assistant Professor of Internal Medicine, Division of Metabolism, Endocrinology and Diabetes, University of Michigan Hospital and Health Systems, Ann Arbor, Michigan

LAURA A. SCHAAP, PhD
Assistant Professor, Department of Health Sciences, Faculty of Earth and Life Sciences, VU University Amsterdam, Amsterdam, The Netherlands

ELSA S. STROTMEYER, PhD, MPH
Assistant Professor, Center for Aging and Population Health, Department of Epidemiology, Graduate School of Public Health, University of Pittsburgh, Pittsburgh, Pennsylvania

ALLYN M. SUSKO, PT, DPT
PhD Candidate, Department of Physical Therapy, School of Health and Rehabilitation Sciences, University of Pittsburgh, Pittsburgh, Pennsylvania

FREDERICO G.S. TOLEDO, MD
Assistant Professor, Division of Endocrinology and Metabolism, Department of Medicine, University of Pittsburgh, Pittsburgh, Pennsylvania

AARON I. VINIK, MD, PhD
Strelitz Diabetes Center, Eastern Virginia Medical School, Norfolk, Virginia

ETTA J. VINIK, MA(Ed)
Strelitz Diabetes Center, Eastern Virginia Medical School, Norfolk, Virginia

STEFANO VOLPATO, MD, MPH
Section of Internal Medicine, Gerontology and Clinical, Nutrition, Department of Medical Sciences, Azienda Ospedaliero-Universitaria di Ferrara U.O. Medicina Interna Universitaria, University of Ferrara, Ferrara, Italy

RACHEL A. WHITMER, PhD
Senior Research Scientist, Epidemiology, Etiology & Prevention, Kaiser Permanente Division of Research, Oakland, California

KRISTINE YAFFE, MD
Vice Chair for Research, Scola Endowed Professor, Departments of Psychiatry, Neurology, and Epidemiology and Biostatistics, University of California, San Francisco; Physician, San Francisco Veterans Affairs Medical Center, San Francisco, California

JANICE C. ZGIBOR, RPh, PhD
Associate Professor of Epidemiology; Assistant Professor of Medicine, and Clinical and Translational Science; Associate Director, Center for Aging and Population Health, Prevention Research Center, Department of Epidemiology, Graduate School of Public Health, University of Pittsburgh, Pittsburgh, Pennsylvania

Contents

focusing on observational studies. Studies show that type 2 diabetes is associated with an unfavorable body composition characterized by more visceral fat, less thigh subcutaneous fat, and more fat infiltration in the muscle compared with persons without the disease. Longitudinal studies found an accelerated decline in muscle mass in older persons with type 2 diabetes. Studies are needed to examine the consequences of these changes in body composition on physical functioning, morbidity, and mortality risk.

Functional decline and physical disability are an important clinical and public health problem in older adults because they are associated with loss of independence, nursing home admission, and mortality. Several impairments and comorbidities related to or associated with diabetes are potential disabling conditions that could account for the excess risk of disability. But in most studies, no single condition explains this association. Accelerated loss of muscle strength is a potential mediator in the disabling effect of diabetes. Because some diabetes-related comorbidities are potential modifiable risk factors, preventing and reducing the excess risk of disability associated with diabetes needs further study.

Osteoarthritis (OA) and type 2 diabetes mellitus (T2DM) often coexist in older adults. Those with T2DM are more susceptible to developing arthritis, which has been traditionally attributed to common risk factors, namely, age and obesity. Alterations in lipid metabolism and hyperglycemia might directly impact cartilage health and subchondral bone, contributing to the development/progression of OA. Adequate management of older persons with both conditions benefits from a comprehensive understanding of the associated risk factors. Common risk factors and emerging links between OA and T2DM are discussed, emphasizing the importance of physical activity and the implications of safe and effective physical activity.

Falls are a major health issue for older adults, especially for those who develop type 2 diabetes who must contend with age-related declines in balance, muscle strength, and walking ability. They must also contend with health-related issues specific to the disease process. Given the general association between these variables and falls, being able to identify which measures negatively impact on balance in older diabetic persons is a critical step. Moreover, designing specific interventions to target these physiologic functions underlying balance and gait control will produce the greatest benefit for reducing falls in older persons with diabetes.

x

Diabetes and Aging
CLINICS IN GERIATRIC MEDICINE

Preface

Diabetes and Aging

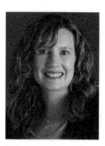

Elsa S. Strotmeyer, PhD, MPH
Editor

> *It takes courage to grow up and be who you really are.*
> —*E.E. Cummings*

Aging with diabetes certainly takes a large amount of courage, and individuals with diabetes need much support to address the many potential complications and conditions associated with disease as they age. As clinicians and researchers, we should strive to address the full scope of the condition. As with Cummings' work, we may need to embrace an unconventional approach. Diabetes is clearly a complex disease in older adults, and this issue will focus on many important conditions surrounding aging with diabetes, which are above and beyond the traditional complications of the disease.

I thank the authors of the reviews for their comprehensive and outstanding contributions on these timely topics. I express a great appreciation to Bridget Leyland, MPH, for her research assistance and organization of the articles, to Jessica McCool and Yonah Korngold, the editors at the *Clinics in Geriatric Medicine*, for their excellent editorial assistance in finalizing the issue, and to Janice Zgibor, RPh, PhD, for her perspectives and contributions to the Introduction. This issue is dedicated to those individuals living and aging with diabetes, particularly within my family. I hope this issue on Diabetes and Aging raises awareness about the scope of geriatric conditions beyond the classic perspectives on diabetes complications.

Elsa S. Strotmeyer, PhD, MPH
Center for Aging and Population Health
Department of Epidemiology
Graduate School of Public Health
University of Pittsburgh
130 N Bellefield Avenue, Room 515
Pittsburgh, PA 15213, USA

E-mail address:
StrotmeyerE@edc.pitt.edu

Clin Geriatr Med 31 (2015) xi
http://dx.doi.org/10.1016/j.cger.2014.09.004
0749-0690/15/$ – see front matter © 2015 Elsevier Inc. All rights reserved.

geriatric.theclinics.com

Introduction

Diabetes and Aging

A critical need exists to more fully address geriatric conditions and related outcomes in diabetes. Currently, 30% of older adults meet the criteria for diabetes diagnosis,[1,2] and a 4.5-fold increase in those aged 65 years and older with diabetes has been projected from 2005 to 2050.[3,4] In this issue, we address the next frontier in treating diabetes by focusing on the following prevalent geriatric conditions and outcomes that disproportionately affect older adults with diabetes: obesity and body composition changes, polypharmacy, atherosclerotic cardiovascular disease, physical function limitations and disability, osteoarthritis, falling, depression, poor cognition, and obstructive sleep apnea. Professional groups, such as the American Geriatric Society (AGS), the American Diabetes Association (ADA), and the European Diabetes Working Party for Older People, have recently acknowledged the issues surrounding older adults with diabetes, and several have graded current evidence for diabetes management.[5–7] However, the guidelines are often vague and discretionary.[8] Evidence-based recommendations for treating clinically complex older adults with diabetes are lacking, particularly for those aged 80 years and older, which are the fastest growing segment of the population.[9,10]

The epidemiology of traditional diabetes complications (eg, cardiovascular disease, neuropathy, etc.) is well-described[5] and has been reviewed by the *Clinics in Geriatric Medicine* previously.[11] In 2008, the highest incidence rates for most diabetes complications were in those aged 75 years and older, followed by the 65 to 75-year-old group, and with lowest rates in those aged 35 to 64.[12] Incidence rates for end-stage renal disease in diabetes were similar among those aged 65 to 74 (319.7/100,000) and 75 years and older (317.7/100,000), but more than double the rate of those aged less than 45 years (151.1/100,000).[12] Furthermore, those aged 75 years and older were approximately twice as likely to visit the emergency department compared with younger age groups with diabetes.[12]

Risk factor control is essential for the prevention of diabetes complications. The proportion of United States adults with diabetes meeting the guidelines for control of risk factors such as glycemia, blood pressure, and lipid levels is between 33% and 49%.[13] For diabetes management in older adults, three primary classifications of health status exist to guide treatment goals: (1) those that are relatively healthy; (2) those with complex medical histories where self-care may be difficult; and (3) those with significant comorbid illness and functional impairment.[6] Recommendations have been made suggesting that older adults with diabetes and life expectancy of less than 2 to 3 years do not have risk reduction of macrovascular complications with management of blood pressure or lipid levels within guidelines and those with life expectancy of less than 5 or 8 years do not have risk reduction of complications or, specifically microvascular disease, respectively, with strict glycemic control.[14] However, life expectancy is challenging to predict so many years in advance. The Health and Retirement Survey, a large, nationally representative sample of older adults in the United States, found that those with diabetes that are relatively healthy and even those with

Clin Geriatr Med 31 (2015) xiii–xvi
http://dx.doi.org/10.1016/j.cger.2014.10.001
0749-0690/15/$ – see front matter © 2015 Published by Elsevier Inc.

geriatric.theclinics.com

self-management difficulty have 91% and 79% respective 5-year survival probabilities and likely would benefit from diabetes management.[15,16] In fact, for all age groups and health status groups, survival probabilities were greater than 50% with the exception of those aged 76 years and older with either dementia, two or more activities of daily living impairments, or long-term residence in a nursing facility.[15,16]

Despite the increased morbidity and mortality with diabetes that exist,[5] great strides have been made in reducing traditional diabetes complications in recent decades. Trends show improvement in control of risk factors, such as glycemia, blood pressure, and lipid levels,[13,17] particularly evident in older age groups, and decreased overall mortality rates,[18,19] even though these are still elevated compared with adults without diabetes. These trends indicate the time has arrived to put a greater focus on geriatric conditions and outcomes in diabetes.

Treatment of diabetes in older adults requires special consideration given the high likelihood of multiple comorbid conditions and potential alterations in metabolism requiring dosage adjustments. In addition to disability in activities of daily living (see Table 1 in the article by de Rekeneire and colleagues elsewhere in this issue) and mobility limitation that are higher among older versus younger adults with diabetes,[12] many older adults have vision, hearing, or manual dexterity issues that may decrease their ability to follow complex dosage regimens or self-management plans. Older adults with diabetes take many medications[20] requiring vigilance for the individual with diabetes and their caregivers (see the article by Peron and colleagues elsewhere in this issue). Shared decision-making with the patient, the patient's family, and caregivers is also important. Providers' concern for overtreatment may result in undertreatment of diabetes and other risk factors for diabetes complications. Therefore, patient-centered, individualized medication regimens need to consider cognitive status, life expectancy, risk for hypoglycemia, and the presence of comorbid conditions or complications.

Current guidelines for diabetes treatment do stress the patient-centered approach;[21,22] however, the scarcity of data from clinical trials in older adults limits an evidence-based approach to treatment. In addition, guidelines are disease-focused and provide little guidance on prioritization or coordination of treatment for those with multiple chronic conditions.[23,24] Hypoglycemia is necessary to consider, whether recognized or unrecognized.[25] For example, hypoglycemia may increase the risk of falls and fall injuries (see the article by Vinik and colleagues elsewhere in this issue). Strategies such as less strict A1C goals and insulin analogue therapies may assist in improving overall glycemic control and in decreasing the risk of hypoglycemia.[25] Clearly, safe and effective treatment approaches are necessary to increase adherence, effectiveness, and promote prevention of diabetes-related conditions and outcomes in the growing cohort of older adults with diabetes.

The geriatric conditions and outcomes reviewed in this issue were selected because of the potential to incorporate evaluation, prevention, and treatment of these comorbidities into common clinical practice, with the goal of improving the health and quality of life for older adults with diabetes. Fracture is one example of a geriatric outcome that is now widely accepted to have a higher risk in diabetes.[26–28] This evidence on higher fracture risk has resulted in current ADA recommendations to assess "fracture history and risk factors in older patients with diabetes and recommend BMD testing if appropriate for the patient's age and sex."[5] In addition to fracture, several current guidelines also note depression, cognitive impairment, obstructive sleep apnea, fatty liver disease, cancer, low testosterone in men, periodontal disease, hearing impairments, and falls as common comorbid conditions with a grade B rating, which is secondary to the strongest A rating for evidence based on "large well-designed clinical trials or well-done meta-analyses."[5,7,29] This issue on Diabetes and Aging addresses several of these plus other common comorbidities that warrant similar initiatives and recommendations. As our population ages with a tremendous burden of diabetes, future directions may include improved and more specific recommendations by relevant professional organizations and well-designed studies to address remaining questions with strong clinical evidence.

Elsa S. Strotmeyer, PhD, MPH
Center for Aging and Population Health
Department of Epidemiology
Graduate School of Public Health
University of Pittsburgh
130 North Bellefield Avenue, Room 515
Pittsburgh, PA 15213, USA

Janice C. Zgibor, RPh, PhD
Center for Aging and Population Health
Prevention Research Center
Department of Epidemiology
Graduate School of Public Health
University of Pittsburgh
130 North Bellefield Avenue, Room 307
Pittsburgh, PA 15213, USA

E-mail addresses:
StrotmeyerE@edc.pitt.edu (E.S. Strotmeyer)
edcjan@pitt.edu (J.C. Zgibor)

REFERENCES

1. Cowie CC, Rust KF, Ford ES, et al. Full accounting of diabetes and pre-diabetes in the U.S. population in 1988-1994 and 2005-2006. Diabetes Care 2009;32:287–94.
2. Kirkman MS, Briscoe VJ, Clark N, et al. Diabetes in older adults. Diabetes Care 2012;35(12):2650–64.
3. Narayan KM, Boyle JP, Geiss LS, et al. Impact of recent increase in incidence on future diabetes burden: U.S., 2005-2050. Diabetes Care 2006;29(9):2114–6.
4. Halter JB. Diabetes mellitus in an aging population: the challenge ahead. J Gerontol A Biol Sci Med Sci 2012;67(12):1297–9.
5. American Diabetes Association. Standards of medical care in diabetes–2014. Diabetes Care 2014;37(Suppl 1):S14–80.
6. Kirkman MS, Briscoe VJ, Clark N, et al. Diabetes in older adults: a consensus report. J Am Geriatr Soc 2012;60(12):2342–56.
7. Sinclair AJ, Paolisso G, Castro M, et al. European Diabetes Working Party for Older People 2011 clinical guidelines for type 2 diabetes mellitus. Executive summary. Diabetes Metab 2011;37(Suppl 3):S27–38. http://dx.doi.org/10.1016/S1262-3636(11)70962-4.
8. Mutasingwa DR, Ge H, Upshur RE. How applicable are clinical practice guidelines to elderly patients with comorbidities? Can Fam Physician 2011;57(7):e253–62.
9. United Nations Department of Economic and Social Affairs. World Population Prospects: The 2012 Revision. Available at: http://esa.un.org/unpd/wpp/. Accessed August 27, 2014.
10. Kinsella K, He W. U.S. Census Bureau, International Population Reports, P95/09-1, An Aging World: 2008. Washington, DC: U.S. Government Printing Office;

2009. Available at. http://www.census.gov/prod/2009pubs/p95-09-1.pdf. Accessed August 27, 2014.

11. Morley JE. Diabetes. Clin Geriatr Med 2008;24(3):395–572.

12. Centers for Disease Control and Prevention. Diabetes Complications. Available at: http://www.cdc.gov/diabetes/statistics/complications_national.htm. Accessed July 29, 2014.

13. Ali MK, Bullard KM, Saaddine JB, et al. Achievement of goals in U.S. diabetes care, 1999-2010. N Engl J Med 2013;368(17):1613–24.

14. Yourman LC, Lee SJ, Schonberg MA, et al. Prognostic indices for older adults: a systematic review. JAMA 2012;307(2):182–92.

15. Blaum C, Cigolle CT, Boyd C, et al. Clinical complexity in middle-aged and older adults with diabetes: the Health and Retirement Study. Med Care 2010;48(4):327–34.

16. Cigolle CT, Kabeto M, Lee P, et al. Clinical complexity and mortality in middle-aged and older adults with diabetes. J Gerontol A Biol Sci Med Sci 2012;67(12):1313–20.

17. Stark Casagrande S, Fradkin JE, Saydah SH, et al. The prevalence of meeting A1C, blood pressure, and LDL goals among people with diabetes, 1988-2010. Diabetes Care 2013;36(8):2271–9.

18. Khalil AC, Roussel R, Mohammedi K, et al. Cause-specific mortality in diabetes: recent changes in trend mortality. Eur J Prev Cardiol 2012;19(3):374–81.

19. Gregg EW, Cheng YJ, Saydah S, et al. Trends in death rates among U.S. adults with and without diabetes between 1997 and 2006: findings from the National Health Interview Survey. Diabetes Care 2012;35(6):1252–7.

20. Grant RW, Devita NG, Singer DE, et al. Polypharmacy and medication adherence in patients with type 2 diabetes. Diabetes Care 2003;26(5):1408–12.

21. Spain M, Edlund BJ. Introducing insulin into diabetes management: transition strategies for older adults. J Gerontol Nurs 2011;37(4):10–5.

22. Inzucchi SE, Bergenstal RM, Buse JB, et al. Management of hyperglycemia in type 2 diabetes: a patient-centered approach: position statement of the American Diabetes Association (ADA) and the European Association for the Study of Diabetes (EASD). Diabetes Care 2012;35(6):1364–79 [Erratum in: Diabetes Care 2013;36(2):490].

23. Pratley RE, Gilbert M. Clinical management of elderly patients with type 2 diabetes mellitus. Postgrad Med 2012;124(1):133–43.

24. Lee PG, Cigolle C, Blaum C. The co-occurrence of chronic diseases and geriatric syndromes: the health and retirement study. J Am Geriatr Soc 2009;57(3):511–6.

25. Zettervall DK. Management of the patient with advanced complications, functional decline, and persistent hyperglycemia. Consult Pharm 2010;25(Suppl B):5–10.

26. Vestergaard P. Discrepancies in bone mineral density and fracture risk in patients with type 1 and type 2 diabetes–a meta-analysis. Osteoporos Int 2007;18(4):427–44.

27. Janghorbani M, Van Dam RM, Willett WC, et al. Systematic review of type 1 and type 2 diabetes mellitus and risk of fracture. Am J Epidemiol 2007;166(5):495–505.

28. Schwartz AV, Vittinghoff E, Bauer DC, et al, for the Study of Osteoporotic Fractures (SOF) Research Group, Osteoporotic Fractures in Men (MrOS) Research Group, Health, Aging, and Body Composition (Health ABC) Research Group. Association of BMD and FRAX score with risk of fracture in older adults with type 2 diabetes. JAMA 2011;305(21):2184–92.

29. American Diabetes Association. Introduction. Diabetes Care 2014;37(Suppl 1):S2–3.

Obesity and Diabetes in an Aging Population

Time to Rethink Definitions and Management?

Amy E. Rothberg, MD, PhD[a],*, Jeffrey B. Halter, MD[b]

KEYWORDS

- Elderly population • Diabetes • Prediabetes • Obesity • Heterogeneous
- Lifestyle interventions

KEY POINTS

- Establishing a diagnosis of prediabetes or diabetes in an elderly population may require more than 1 measure of glycemia.
- The geriatric population represents a heterogeneous group of individuals in whom vigilance and a tailored approach are warranted.
- Management of diabetes in an elderly population requires examining each patient's comorbid conditions, functional status, life expectancy, and preferences.
- Obesity is highly prevalent. Older individuals benefit as much as, or to a greater degree, from intensive lifestyle interventions to reduce weight compared with younger obese individuals.

INTRODUCTION

Diabetes mellitus (DM) represents a group of disorders characterized by hyperglycemia; microvascular complications including retinopathy, nephropathy, and peripheral neuropathy; and an increased risk of cardiovascular disease. The diagnosis of diabetes is based on fasting and post–glucose load blood glucose thresholds. The

Disclosures: A.E. Rothberg reports consulting with Novo Nordisk outside the submitted work. J.B. Halter reports consulting with Sanofi and with Boehringer Ingelheim outside the submitted work.
Funding: A.E. Rothberg reports funding from BCBSM (1835.PIRAP), Michigan Institute for Clinical Research (2UL1TR00433), and National Institutes of Health (P30 DK089503-01). J.B. Halter reports grants from the John A. Hartford Foundation, National Institutes of Health, National Institute on Aging (AG024824 and AG040938), and Alliance for Academic Internal Medicine.
[a] Division of Metabolism, Endocrinology and Diabetes, University of Michigan Hospital and Health Systems, Domino's Farms, Lobby G, Suite 1500, 24 Frank Lloyd Wright Drive, Ann Arbor, MI 48106, USA; [b] Division of Geriatric and Palliative Medicine, University of Michigan Geriatrics Center, 300 North Ingalls, Room 901, Ann Arbor, MI 48109-2007, USA
* Corresponding author.
E-mail address: arothber@umich.edu

most recent American Diabetes Association (ADA) criteria for the diagnosis of diabetes and prediabetes are summarized in **Box 1**.[1]

However, glucose levels in the population are a continuum. Therefore, these diagnostic criteria to distinguish between normal and diabetic levels are arbitrary. Glucose levels are also used to define prediabetes (ie, impaired fasting glucose and impaired glucose tolerance).

More than 30% of older adults in the United States meet these ADA criteria for diabetes,[2,3] and approximately 40% of people with a known diagnosis of diabetes are older than 65 years.[2] The number of people more than 65 years of age with diabetes is projected to increase by 4.5-fold between 2005 and 2050.[4,5] Because many other older people meet ADA criteria for prediabetes, less than 30% of the US population more than 65 years of age have normal glucose levels.[2]

The glucose cutoffs for diabetes and prediabetes were selected because of predictions of increased risk of microvascular and neuropathic complications. Progressively higher glucose levels from the normal to the prediabetic to the diabetic range are associated with a progressively higher risk of cardiovascular disease, as shown in **Fig. 1**.[6–9]

However, for individuals who meet criteria for prediabetes but not diabetes, the risk may be modest and hard to separate from overlap with the other components of metabolic syndrome (obesity, low high-density lipoprotein level, high triglyceride levels, and increased blood pressure).[10,11] None of these criteria make adjustments for age, because these cutoffs predict risk for diabetes complications in all age groups.

Recent changes to the diagnostic criteria for prediabetes and diabetes include the addition of hemoglobin A1c (HbA1c) (see **Box 1**),[1] which also predicts microvascular complications. Advantages to HbA1c as a diagnostic test compared with glucose measurements include convenience (it can be obtained at any time of day and without regard to caloric intake), less day-to-day variability, and international standardization of the assay. However, there are many situations in which HbA1c does not accurately

---

Box 1
ADA criteria for the diagnosis of diabetes and prediabetes

Criteria for the diagnosis of diabetes: 4 options

Hemoglobin A1c (HbA1c) level greater than or equal to 6.5%[a]

    Performed in a laboratory using National Glycohemoglobin Standardization Program (NGSP)-certified method standardized to The Diabetes Control and Complications Trial (DCCT) assay

Fasting plasma glucose (FPG) greater than or equal to 126 mg/dL (7.0 mmol/L)[a]

    Fasting defined as no caloric intake for greater than or equal to 8 and less than or equal to 12 hours

Two-hour post glucola (PG) greater than or equal to 200 mg/dL (11.1 mmol/L) during OGTT (75 g)[a]

Random PG greater than or equal to 200 mg/dL (11.1 mmol/L)

    In persons with symptoms of hyperglycemia or hyperglycemic crisis

Criteria for the diagnosis of prediabetes: 3 options

HbA1c level 5.7% to 6.4%

FPG 100 to 125 mg/dL

Two-hour PG 140 to 199 mg/dL during oral glucose tolerance testing (OGTT) (75 g)

    [a] In the absence of unequivocal hyperglycemia, results should be confirmed using repeat testing.

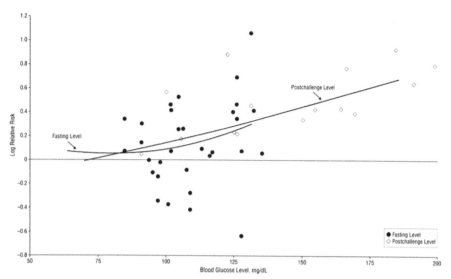

Fig. 1. Dose-response relationship of cardiovascular disease with fasting and postchallenge blood glucose levels. To convert glucose to millimoles per liter, multiply by 0.0555. (*From* Levitan ED, Song Y, Ford ES, et al. Is nondiabetic hyperglycemia a risk factor for cardiovascular disease? A meta-analysis of prospective studies. Arch Intern Med 2004;164(19):2147–55. Copyright © 2004 American Medical Association. All rights reserved.)

reflect mean glucose concentrations. Because HbA1c depends on the circulating life span of red blood cells, any condition affecting the red blood cell turnover affects HbA1c independently of glucose level. HbA1c cannot be used for diabetes diagnosis in the presence of hemoglobinopathies, hemolysis, acute bleeding, transfusion, iron-deficiency anemia, erythropoietin therapy, or severe chronic diseases (eg, chronic kidney or liver disease). HbA1c levels have been reported to be higher among US racial and ethnic minority populations than among white people, independently of glycemia.[12,13] Further, HBA1c has been shown to be positively associated with the total level of fat intake.[14]

Both glucose levels and HbA1c may have additional limitations in the elderly population. To a small extent, fasting glucose levels, and to a larger extent postchallenge glucose levels, increase as people age. A cross-sectional analysis in adults without known diabetes in the Screening for Impaired Glucose Tolerance (SIGT) study 2005 to 2008 (n = 1573) and the National Health and Nutrition Examination Survey (NHANES) 2005 to 2006 (n = 1184) showed that HbA1c levels increased 0.87 mmol/mol (0.08%) per 10 years in subjects without diabetes, and 0.76 mmol/mol (0.07%) per 10 years in subjects with normal glucose tolerance (all P<.001).[15] In both datasets, the HbA1c level of an 80-year-old individual with normal glucose tolerance would be 3.82 mmol/mol (0.35%) greater than that of a 30-year-old with normal glucose tolerance; a difference that is clinically significant. Moreover, the specificity of HbA1c-based diagnostic criteria for prediabetes decreased substantially with increasing age.[15] NHANES II showed a 7-mg/dL increase, per decade of life, in plasma glucose 2 hours after a 75-g oral glucose load.[15] In an analysis of individuals in the Baltimore Longitudinal Study of Aging, age had an independent effect on glucose tolerance, even after adjusting for adiposity, fat distribution, and fitness. In contrast, these indices did account for the decline in glucose tolerance among young and middle-aged adults.[16] Hence, when the diagnostic criteria include the 2-hour post–glucose challenge glucose level, ascertainment of diabetes is more complete in the elderly population than when the diagnosis is based on fasting plasma glucose (FPG) level alone.[3,15,16]

A more troubling problem is that HbA1c levels seem to increase with age independently of mean glycemia. Pani and colleagues[17] examined the relationship between age and HbA1c in the nondiabetic population included in the Framingham Offspring Study and the NHANES 2001 to 2004. In multivariate analysis adjusting for sex, FPG, and 2-hour post–glucose load glucose level, HbA1c level still increased with age. Lipska and colleagues[18] examined the performance of HbA1c compared with FPG in diagnosing diabetes and prediabetes, per ADA criteria, in older adults. Between the ages of 70 and 79 years and in black compared with white people, sensitivity and specificity of HbA1c were 57% and 98% for diabetes and 47% and 85% for prediabetes, respectively. The HbA1c values meeting ADA criteria agreed closely with glucose cutoffs for these diagnoses. However, many more people met diagnostic criteria based on glucose values than HbA1c in this population. Older Americans identified with diabetes and, to a lesser extent, prediabetes from HbA1c were more likely to be female and black than those identified by FPG criteria.

Although there may be a subset of elderly individuals identified by either FPG or HbA1c, the identification of prediabetes or diabetes in the elderly population may need to rely on both measures.

Glycemic Management

Recommendations on the management of diabetes in adults aged 65 years or older were articulated in an ADA consensus report published in December 2012.[3] This report recognized the heterogeneity of the elderly diabetes population and emphasized individualized targets for glycemia, blood pressure, and dyslipidemia based on health status, number of comorbid health conditions, life expectancy, and the existence of cognitive impairment. Thus, providers should actively engage their patients in shared decision making with respect to their treatment preferences, ability for self-management, and treatment targets, and stratify patients by their likelihood of risk and benefit from intensive therapies.[19,20] If goals are not being met, patients should be reevaluated to determine the contributing causes and the patient's understanding, adherence, and motivation. Therapeutic targets may need to be adjusted.

Evidence from the United Kingdom Prospective Diabetes Study (UKPDS), a randomized controlled trial of middle-aged adults with incident type 2 DM (T2DM) and few comorbidities, showed that a 1% reduction in HbA1c translated to a 37% reduction in microvascular outcomes and a 21% reduction in any diabetes-related end point.[21] Despite an early loss of glycemic differences, a continued reduction in microvascular risk and emergent risk reductions for myocardial infarction and death from any cause were observed during 10 years of posttrial follow-up. Therefore, the benefits of early intensive therapy persisted for 10 years or more of follow-up when the population was reaching ages of late 60s and 70s. More recent trials including patients up to age 75 years have failed to show reduction of cardiovascular outcomes with intensification of glucose level–lowering therapy.[22–24] Although the Action to Control Cardiovascular Risk in Diabetes (ACCORD) trial was stopped early because of excessive mortality in the intensive therapy arm, this excessive mortality was primarily among participants younger than 65 years.[22] However, age was a risk factor for severe hypoglycemia in ACCORD.[25]

Furthermore, research is lacking regarding the benefit of tight glucose control in the oldest age group (>80 years). Intensive glycemic and other risk factor controls may not be pragmatic or responsible in those who have underlying complicating medical conditions, because of risk of hypoglycemia, polypharmacy, and drug-disease interactions. Vijan and colleagues[26] examined the effect of patients' risks and preferences on health gain or disutility with plasma glucose level lowering. Using a Markov model, they showed that, once moderate control of HbA1c level (9%) was achieved, patients' views of the burdens of treatment were the most important factor in the net benefit of glucose level–lowering treatments.

Diabetes is associated with lower levels of cognitive functioning[27,28] and greater cognitive decline,[29,30] which pose a greater risk of hypoglycemia.[31] Elderly patients may experience impaired awareness of the autonomic warning symptoms of hypoglycemia secondary to diminished or altered counter-regulation, and further may have a diminished capacity or delayed response to intervene[32,33] (discussed further by Mayeda and colleagues elsewhere in this issue).

A central concept in geriatric diabetes care guidelines is that providers should base decisions regarding treatment targets on health status and life expectancy, as suggested in **Table 1**.[3] This framework is based on the work of Blaum and colleagues,[34] which identified 3 major classes of older patients with diabetes from the Health and Retirement Study (HRS) of the US population aged 51 years and older, based on health status defined by the presence and number of comorbidities or impairments in functional status. Patients whose life expectancy is limited (eg, <5 years, <10 years) are considered unlikely to benefit from intensive glucose control; therefore, guidelines suggest less intensive management.[1,35,36] In contrast, those with longer life expectancy may be appropriate candidates for more intensive intervention. However, average remaining life expectancy, although shorter with increasing population age, is difficult to predict for an individual.[37,38] Furthermore, a longitudinal study of mortality in adults with diabetes in the HRS found that 5-year survival probabilities were good: 91% in the healthiest people with diabetes, 79% in people with modest comorbidities, and still more than 50% in people with substantial comorbidities and disabilities.[38]

Table 1
A framework for considering treatment goals for glycemia in older adults with diabetes

Health Status	Rationale	Reasonable HbA1c Goal (%)	FPG or Preprandial Glucose (mg/dL)	Bedtime Glucose (mg/dL)
Healthy	Longer life expectancy	<7.5	90–130	90–150
Complex intermediate	Intermediate life expectancy; high treatment burden; hypoglycemia vulnerability; fall risk	~8.0	90–150	100–180
Very complex Poor health	Limited life expectancy; treatment benefit uncertain	~8.5	100–180	110–200

Healthy: few coexisting chronic illnesses, intact cognitive and functional status. Complex/intermediate health: multiple coexisting chronic illnesses, impairment in 2 or more instrumental activities of daily living (ADL), or mild to moderate cognitive impairment. Very complex/poor health: long-term care, end-stage chronic illness, moderate to severe cognitive impairment, or 2 or more ADL dependencies.

Data from Kirkman MS, Briscoe VJ, Clark N, et al. Consensus report: diabetes in older adults. Diabetes Care 2012;35(12):2650–64.

Only people with substantial comorbidities and disabilities who were more than 76 years of age had a 5-year survival rate less than 50%. Thus, there remains a substantial challenge to identify those patients with diabetes whose likelihood of long-term survival is so low that prevention efforts are no longer warranted.

As not every patient is clearly in a particular category, consideration of patient/caregiver preferences is an important aspect of treatment individualization. In addition, patients' health statuses and preferences may change over time and therefore treatment goals may need to be modified.[39,40] Greater latitude to treatment targets for those in the poorest of health and/or with a history of hypoglycemia may be taken; limiting exposure to severe hyperglycemia and its attendant risks is indicated for most patients. A provider should forge a secure therapeutic alliance with the patient to reduce both the burden of diabetes on the patient and the economic burden of diabetes on the health system.

In addition to issues related to glycemia, other modifiable cardiometabolic risk factors including overweight/obesity, blood pressure control, and lipids need to be considered in diabetes management. However, this discussion focuses on obesity and its management, in relation to diabetes prevention and treatment.

Role of Obesity in the Development and Prevention of Diabetes in an Elderly Population

In the US population, the prevalence of obesity has increased from around 15% between the 1960s and 1980s to 34% between 2007 and 2008 (**Fig. 2**).[41] Elderly individuals represent 12% to 15% of the general population, with projections estimating this proportion to represent 20% to 25% by the year 2030. By 2050, the number of older adults, defined as persons aged 65 years and older, is expected to more than double; from 40.2 million to 88.5 million. At present, more than one-third of US adults aged 65

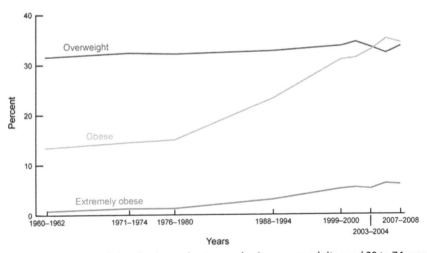

Fig. 2. Trends in overweight, obesity, and extreme obesity among adults aged 20 to 74 years: United States, 1960 to 2008. Overweight is defined as a body mass index (BMI) of greater than or equal to 25 kg/m², but less than 30 kg/m²; obesity is defined as a BMI greater than or equal to 30 kg/m² but less than 40 kg/m²; extreme obesity is defined as a BMI greater than or equal to 40 kg/m². (*From* CDC/NCHS. National Health Examination Survey cycle 1 (1960–1962); and National Health and Nutrition Examination Survey 1 (1971–1974), II (1976–1980), and III (1988–2000, 2001–2002, 2003–2004, 2005–2006, and 2007–2008).)

years and older is obese as defined by a body mass index (BMI) greater than or equal to 30 kg/m^2 (US Centers for Disease Control and Prevention [CDC]). Obesity is more common among people aged 65 to 74 years compared with those aged 75 years and older for both men and women, as shown in **Fig. 3**, reflecting changes in not only body weight but body composition.[42]

In the United States, obesity has surpassed smoking as the leading cause of preventable death and may be responsible for 6% to 10% of national health care expenditures. Medicare spending has grown about 9-fold in the past 25 years, increasing from $37 billion in 1980 to $336 billion in 2005. The direct medical costs related to all obesity are estimated to be $191 billion annually.[43] Prediabetes and diabetes are important consequences of obesity and parallel the trends in obesity prevalence. The direct medical costs attributable to diagnosed diabetes in 2012 (ADA) were $306 billion. For all of these reasons, finding and implementing effective interventions to prevent or treat obesity is a national priority and should not exclude an older population based on expectations of limited effect or impact on mortality.

Over the past 2 decades, the rate of obesity among elderly individuals has increased dramatically independently of sex, race, and educational level. Excess weight may disproportionately affect the health status of older adults by contributing to illness, impairments, poor quality of life, functional decline, disability, and death. The criterion to define obesity (ie, based on BMI) is only a surrogate measure of body fat. The association between BMI and all-cause mortality is J shaped, with normal or healthy weight defined as a BMI between 18.5 and 24.9 kg/m^2, which represents the lowest risk.[44] Defining a healthy weight in older adults poses unique challenges because of important physiologic changes related to aging (ie, changes in body composition and stature).[45] The current World Health Organization cutoffs may not be appropriate in this population. Systematic review of ~26 cohort studies of healthy elderly people found a similar mortality risk in the overweight elderly (BMI, 25–29.8 kg/m^2) compared with those with BMIs of 18.5 to 24.9.[46] In contrast, some other large prospective cohort studies have reported an increased mortality risk in elderly people with BMIs less than 22 kg/m^2.[47]

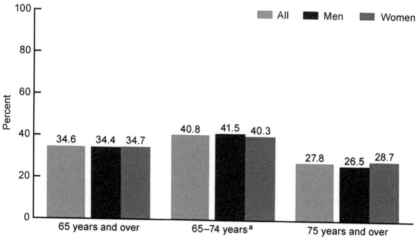

Fig. 3. Prevalence of obesity among adults ages 65 years and older, by sex: United States, 2007 to 2010. [a] Significantly different from 75 years and older. (*From* CDC/NCHS. National Health and Nutrition Examination Survey, 2007–2010.)

In cross-sectional studies, body weight seems to progressively increase until the sixth decade of life, remain fairly constant between the ages of 65 and 70 years, and decline thereafter.[48] However, these observations can be affected by survival bias. Obese persons have higher mortality at younger ages.[49] Premature mortality in obese young and middle-aged adults tends to decrease mean body weight and BMI in surviving older adults. Nevertheless, this age-dependent weight loss is characterized by stable or increasing adiposity with redistribution of fat into the visceral and ectopic depots and loss of fat from subcutaneous tissues and a concomitant decline in lean mass[50,51] (discussed in detail by Koster and colleagues elsewhere in this issue). Loss in height is common because of narrowed intervertebral disc spaces and osteoporotic vertebral compression and kyphosis.[45,52] Therefore, BMI may not accurately reflect adiposity, fat distribution, or mortality risk in the elderly population. Other measures to assess body fatness and distribution of fat (such as measuring waist circumference) need to be considered and likely applied more routinely in the geriatric population. This consideration is particularly relevant given the epidemiology of weight-associated cardiometabolic risk factors in this population. Although the protective or nonadverse effect of overweight or obesity in elderly people has been debated, recent data do not confirm an obesity paradox. The absolute mortality risk associated with increased BMI increases with age, up to the age of 75 years, because of the marked increase in mortality with advancing age. Therefore, from a clinical standpoint, the health complications associated with obesity increase linearly with increasing BMI until the age of 75 years.[53]

A host of metabolic and hormonal changes occur in association with increased adiposity, particularly visceral adiposity. Progressive deficits in insulin action or secretion, altered adipokine regulation, altered gut–central nervous system signaling, and increased secretion of proinflammatory cytokines contribute to the evolution of T2DM in individuals who are genetically susceptible to disease.[54,55] All components of the metabolic syndrome (excess abdominal fat, impaired glucose metabolism, dyslipidemia, and high blood pressure) are prevalent in older populations. Moreover, the prevalence of the metabolic syndrome increases with age.[56] The odds of developing the metabolic syndrome in individuals who are greater than or equal to 65 years of age compared with those who are 20 to 34 years of age was 5.8 in men and 4.9 in women. In addition, increased abdominal fat mass is independently associated with the metabolic syndrome in men and women aged 70 to 79 years.[57]

Interventions to Reduce Obesity and Prevent Diabetes: Lifestyle

Studies addressing weight loss in older adults have had conflicting results. Several population studies have evaluated the effect of weight loss on mortality in middle to older age groups.[58–63] Data from most such studies have indicated that weight loss is associated with increased, rather than decreased, mortality. However, none of these studies were randomized controlled trials. Most used self-reported weight change, and did not distinguish between weight loss in obese and lean subjects or between intentional and unintentional weight loss. Nondeliberate weight loss is a common complication of many serious diseases, which could confound the interpretation of weight-loss effects on mortality. In contrast, several studies, conducted primarily in middle-aged persons (aged 40–65 years at baseline), differentiated between the effects of intentional and unintentional weight loss.[62–68] The results from some of these studies are that intentional weight loss was associated with reduced mortalities in persons with diabetes, impaired glucose tolerance, and other weight-related health conditions.[64–68]

Lifestyle interventions, as studied in both the Diabetes Prevention Program (DPP) and the Action for Health in Diabetes Study (Look AHEAD), have conclusively shown meaningful reductions in weight and other comorbid health conditions, as summarized in **Table 2**.[69,70] These interventions translated to even greater improvements in an elderly population,[69–71] refuting the concept that weight loss might negatively affect older individuals, at least among these high-risk subgroups.[72]

The DPP studied more than 3000 individuals greater than or equal to 25 years of age at high risk for T2DM and randomized them to placebo, lifestyle intervention, or metformin. Lifestyle intervention included a deficit in calories of 400 to 500 kcal/d to promote a greater than or equal to 7% weight loss and an increase in physical activity, implemented as brisk walking for greater than or equal to 150 min/wk. Metformin was administered as 850 mg twice daily. Weight loss and risk reduction were greatest among those aged 60 to 85 years at randomization to the lifestyle intervention, with a 71% risk reduction in the progression to diabetes at the end of the randomized trial[72] and a 49% persistent risk reduction at 10 years total follow-up, including 3 years of randomized therapy and 7 years of observational follow-up.[69] Metformin was less effective in this age group. This lack of efficacy in the older populations may be related to changes in muscle metabolism and fat oxidation.

The Look AHEAD study[70,73] assessed the effects of intentional weight loss on cardiovascular outcomes in 5145 overweight/obese adults 45 to 75 years of age with T2DM, who were randomly assigned to intensive lifestyle intervention (ILI) or usual care (ie, diabetes support education). Participants in the ILI were provided with a comprehensive behavioral intervention, expected to induce an average loss greater than or equal to 7% of initial weight. Individual participants were given a goal of losing 10% or more of initial weight in order to increase the likelihood of meeting the 7% study-wide goal. Those in the ILI were asked to reduce their calories to 1200 to 1500 kcal/d (initial weight <114 kg) or 1500 to 1800 kcal/d (initial weight >114 kg). In weeks 3 to 18 of the study, participants were offered a liquid meal replacement

Table 2
Description of the DPP and the Look AHEAD study

Study	Characteristics of Population	Elderly (%)	Lifestyle Intervention Goals	Weight Outcomes (% from Baseline)	Other Health Risk Outcomes
DPP	3234 individuals at high risk for DM based on OGTT	20	≥7% weight loss and ≥150 min of moderate physical activity/wk	5–7	71% reduced risk to progression to DM; 10-y follow-up 49% reduced risk (vs 39% for entire cohort)
Look AHEAD	5145 individuals with T2DM at risk for CV events	17	≥7% weight loss and ≥150–200 min of moderate physical activity/wk	5–10	No change in primary outcome of CV events; improvements in cardiometabolic risk factors

Abbreviations: CV, cardiovascular; T2DM, type 2 DM.
Data from Diabetes Prevention Program Research Group. 10-year follow-up of diabetes incidence and weight loss in the Diabetes Prevention Program Outcomes Study. Lancet 2009;374:1677–86; and Rejeski WJ, Ip EH, Bertoni AG, et al, Look AHEAD Research Group. Lifestyle change and mobility in obese adults with type 2 diabetes. N Engl J Med 2012;366:1209–17.

plan given the evidence that this significantly increased weight loss compared with a self-selected diet with the same calorie goal. There were no adverse outcomes reported with regard to diet. Differences in mean weight loss (%) are reported in **Fig. 4**.[73]

In summary, lifestyle intervention is a feasible and reasonable approach to reduce weight and the complications related to excess weight. Elderly at-risk individuals perform as well and benefit equally or more from these behavioral interventions as younger individuals. Note that weight loss and improved fitness slowed the decline in mobility in overweight adults with T2DM and improved functional status.[70]

Interventions to Reduce Obesity and Prevent Diabetes: Bariatric Surgery

In February 2006, the Centers for Medicare and Medicaid Services (CMS) expanded the national coverage for bariatric surgery procedures for Medicare beneficiaries more than 65 years of age. However, Medicare coverage of weight-loss surgery is decided from region to region and case by case. Beneficiaries are required to receive care in high-volume centers and from qualified surgeons (as certified by the American College of Surgeons or the American Society for Bariatric Surgery); to have a BMI of 35 kg/m^2 or higher; and to have a serious health condition in addition to obesity, such as T2DM, hypertension, or coronary artery disease. The decision also expanded coverage to 3 bariatric surgery procedures: laparoscopic and open Roux-en-Y gastric bypass, laparoscopic adjustable gastric banding, and laparoscopic and open biliopancreatic diversion with duodenal switch. Bariatric surgery, now also termed metabolic surgery, has been shown to improve glycemia and even induce remissions in T2DM, depending on the type of procedure performed; the duration and severity of type 2 DM (T2DM) at the time of surgery; and the length of follow-up.[74] However,

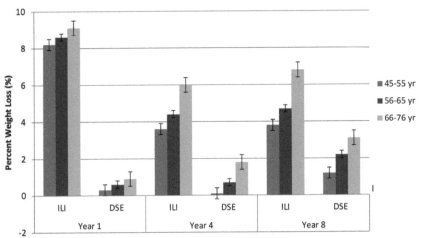

Fig. 4. Eight-year weight loss, by age group, in the Look AHEAD study of people with T2DM. The bars depict mean percent weight loss from initial weight at years 1, 4, and 8 of the study, comparing people randomized to intensive lifestyle intervention (ILI) versus diabetes support and education (DSE). Regardless of age, ILI was more effective than DSE for weight reduction, although the difference between ILI and DSE decreased over time. The greatest weight loss at each time point was for those in the oldest age group, for both ILI and DSE ($P<.017$ for comparison of different age groups). Values shown are means ± standard error of the mean for the intention-to-treat population (total ILI, 2570; DSE, 2575). (*Data from* The Look AHEAD Research Group. Eight-year weight losses with an intensive lifestyle intervention. Obesity (Silver Spring) 2014;22(1):5–13.)

few studies have addressed any of the long-term outcomes, particularly the impact of bariatric surgery on T2DM in the geriatric population.

In a retrospective analysis of Cleveland Clinic data, adjustable gastric banding was the procedure most often offered to older patients with greater morbidities and surgical risk. This restrictive procedure has a much lower rate of biochemical remission rates. Varela and colleagues[74] performed a retrospective review of data obtained from the University Health System Consortium Clinical Data Base for all elderly (>60 years old) and nonelderly (19–60 years old) people who underwent bariatric surgery for the treatment of morbid obesity between 1999 and 2005. Compared with non-elderly patients, elderly patients who underwent bariatric surgery had more comorbidities, longer lengths of stay (4.9 days vs 3.8 days), and more overall complications (19% vs 11%). The in-hospital mortality was also higher in the elderly group (>60 years old; 0.7% vs 0.3%) compared with younger ages. However, when risk adjusted, the observed/expected mortality ratio for the elderly group was 0.9, which was similar between groups. In a subset of elderly patients with a preexisting cardiac condition (n = 236), the in-hospital mortality was 4.7%.[74]

Bariatric surgery in the elderly population represents only a small fraction (~2.7%) of the number of bariatric operations performed at academic centers,[74] so the interpretation and risks are confounded by small numbers. Despite historically small numbers, as in the general population, bariatric surgery is being more widely adopted. Older patients have more preoperative and postoperative comorbidities and greater mortality, and the weight loss is usually less than in younger patients.[75] However, bariatric surgery is considered as safe as other gastrointestinal procedures in elderly, obese patients because the observed mortality is better than the expected (risk-adjusted) mortality.[75]

SUMMARY

Regardless of pathophysiology and diagnostic criteria, the population of older adults with diabetes is highly heterogeneous. As older adults with T2DM age and develop multiple comorbid health conditions, they may experience many challenges to good diabetes care and self-management. Age of diagnosis and duration of diabetes largely determine the likelihood for comorbidity; older adults who have had diabetes for decades are more likely to have developed comorbid health conditions. Concurrent comorbid health conditions are the traditional diabetes complications, which depend on diabetes duration. Discordant comorbidities are non–DM related and are age dependent. Some older patients are newly diagnosed with diabetes and have few other health problems. Others may have cognitive problems, psychological/emotional problems, or physical frailty, and have many functional disabilities. Remaining life expectancies are variable and often difficult to predict. Thus, treating such a diverse elderly population may result in inadequate glycemic control either because of overtreatment, leading to hypoglycemia, or because of other complications and preexisting comorbidities. Therefore, it is imperative that treatment decisions are based on patient preferences, unique and likely evolving health status, and longevity.

REFERENCES

1. American Diabetes Association. Standards of medical care in diabetes—2014. Diabetes Care 2014;37:S14–80. http://dx.doi.org/10.2337/dc14-S014.
2. Cowie CC, Rust KF, Ford ES, et al. Full accounting of diabetes and pre-diabetes in the U.S. population in 1988-1994 and 2005-2006. Diabetes Care 2009;32: 287–94.

3. Kirkman MS, Briscoe VJ, Clark N, et al. Consensus report: diabetes in older adults. Diabetes Care 2012;35(12):2650–64.

4. Narayan KM, Boyle JP, Geiss LS, et al. Impact of recent increase in incidence on future diabetes burden: U.S., 2005-2050. Diabetes Care 2006;29:2114–6. http://dx.doi.org/10.2337/dc06-1136.

5. Halter JB. Guest editorial, diabetes mellitus in an aging population: the challenge ahead. Special issue on glucose homeostasis. J Gerontol A Biol Sci Med Sci 2012;67(12):1297–9.

6. DeFronzo RA. Insulin resistance, lipotoxicity, type 2 diabetes and atherosclerosis: the missing links. The Claude Bernard lecture. Diabetologia 2010;53(7): 1270–87. http://dx.doi.org/10.1007/s00125-010-1684-1.

7. Bornfelt KE, Tabas I. Insulin resistance, hyperglycemia, and atherosclerosis. Cell Metab 2011;14(5):575–85. http://dx.doi.org/10.1016/j.cmet.2011.07.015.

8. Halter JB, Musi N, McFarland Horne F, et al. Diabetes mellitus and cardiovascular disease in older adults: current status and future directions. Diabetes 2014; 63(8):2578–89.

9. Levitan EB, Song Y, Ford ES, et al. Is nondiabetic hyperglycemia a risk factor for cardiovascular disease? A meta-analysis of prospective studies. Arch Intern Med 2004;164(19):2147–55.

10. Grundy SM. Pre-diabetes, metabolic syndrome, and cardiovascular risk. J Am Coll Cardiol 2012;59(7):635–43. http://dx.doi.org/10.1016/j.jacc.2011.08.080.

11. Shaye K, Amir T, Shlomo S, et al. Fasting glucose levels within the high normal range predict cardiovascular outcome. Am Heart J 2012;164(1):111–6. http://dx.doi.org/10.1016/j.ahj.2012.03.023.

12. Cohen RM, Haggerty S, Herman WH. HbA1c for the diagnosis of diabetes and prediabetes: is it time for a mid-course corrections? J Clin Endocrinol Metab 2010;95(12):5203–6.

13. Herman WH, Cohen RM. Racial and ethnic differences in the relationship between HbA1c and blood glucose: implications for the diagnosis of diabetes. J Clin Endocrinol Metab 2012;97(4):1067–72.

14. Harding AH, Sargeant LA, Welch A, et al. Fat consumption and HbA1c levels: the EPIC-Norfolk study. Diabetes Care 2001;24:1911–6.

15. Dubowitz N, Xue W, Long Q, et al. Aging is associated with increased HbA1c levels, independently of glucose levels and insulin resistance, and also with decreased HbA1c diagnostic specificity. Diabet Med 2014;31(8):927–35. http://dx.doi.org/10.1111/dme.12459.

16. Shimokata H, Muller DC, Fleg JL, et al. Age as independent determinant of glucose tolerance. Diabetes 1991;40:44–51. http://dx.doi.org/10.2337/diab. 40.1.44.

17. Pani LK, Meigs JB, Driver C, et al. Effect of aging on a1c levels in individuals without diabetes. Diabetes Care 2008;31:1991–6.

18. Lipska KJ, De Rekeneire N, Van Ness PH, et al. Identifying dysglycemic states in older adults: implications of the emerging use of hemoglobin A1c. J Clin Endocrinol Metab 2010;95(12):5289–95.

19. Barry MJ, Edgman-Levitan S. Shared decision making – pinnacle of patient-centered care. N Engl J Med 2012;366:780–1.

20. Montori VM, Gafni A, Charles C. A shared treatment decision-making approach between patients with chronic conditions and their clinicians: the case of diabetes. Health Expect 2006;9:25–36.

21. Holman RR, Paul SK, Bethel MA, et al. 10-year follow-up of intensive glucose control in type 2 diabetes. N Engl J Med 2008;359(15):1577–89.

22. Gerstein HC, Miller ME, Byington RP, et al. Action to control cardiovascular risk in Diabetes Study Group. Effects of intensive glucose lowering in type 2 diabetes. N Engl J Med 2008;358(24):2545–59.

23. Patel A, MacMahon S, Chalmers J, et al, The ADVANCE Collaborative Group. Intensive blood glucose control and vascular outcomes in patients with type 2 diabetes. N Engl J Med 2008;358(24):2560–72.

24. Duckworth W, Abraira C, Moritz T, et al. Glucose control and vascular complications in veterans with type 2 diabetes. N Engl J Med 2009;360(2):129–39.

25. Miller ME, Bonds DE, Gerstein HC, et al, ACCORD Investigators. The effects of baseline characteristics, glycaemia treatment approach, and glycated haemoglobin concentration on the risk of severe hypoglycaemia: post hoc epidemiological analysis of the ACCORD study. BMJ 2010;340:b5444.

26. Vijan S, Sussman JB, Yudkim JS, et al. Effect of patients' risk and preferences on health gains with plasma glucose level lowering in type 2 diabetes mellitus. JAMA Intern Med 2014. http://dx.doi.org/10.1001/jamainternmed.2014.2894.

27. Exalto LG, Whitmer RA, Kappele LJ, et al. An update on type 2 diabetes, vascular dementia and Alzheimer's disease. Exp Gerontol 2012;47(11):858–64.

28. Bordier L, Doucet J, Boudet J, et al. Update on cognitive decline and dementia in elderly patients with diabetes. Diabetes Metab 2014. http://dx.doi.org/10.1016/j.diabet.2014.02.002.

29. Schnaider Beeri M, Goulbourt U, Silverman JM. Diabetes mellitus in midlife and the risk of dementia three decades later. Neurology 2004;63:1902–7.

30. Xu W, Qiu C, Gatz M, et al. Mid- and late-life diabetes in relation to the risk of dementia: a population-based twin study. Diabetes 2009;58(1):71–7. http://dx.doi.org/10.2337/db08-0586.

31. Punthakee Z, Miller ME, Launer LJ, et al. Poor cognitive function and risk of severe hypoglycemia in type 2 diabetes: post hoc epidemiologic analysis of the ACCORD trial. Diabetes Care 2012;35(4):787–93.

32. Meneilly GS, Tessier D. Diabetes in the elderly. Diabet Med 1995;12(11):949–60.

33. Bremer JP, Jauch-Chara K, Hallschmid M, et al. Hypoglycemia unawareness in older compared with middle-aged patients with type 2 diabetes. Diabetes Care 2009;32(8):1513–7.

34. Blaum C, Cigolle CT, Boyd C, et al. Clinical complexity in middle-aged and older adults with diabetes: the Health and Retirement Study. Med Care 2010;48(4):327–34.

35. California Health Foundation/American Geriatrics Society Panel on Improving Care for Elders with Diabetes. Guidelines for improving the care of the older person with diabetes mellitus. J Am Geriatr Soc 2003;51:S265–80.

36. European Diabetes Working Party for older people 2011: clinical guidelines for type 2 diabetes mellitus. Executive summary. Diabetes Metab 2011;37:S27–38.

37. Huang ES, Zhang Q, Gandra N, et al. The effect of comorbid illness and functional status on the expected benefits of intensive glucose control in order patients with type 2 diabetes: a decision analysis. Ann Intern Med 2008;149:11–20.

38. Yourman LC, Lee SJ, Schonberg MA, et al. Prognostic indices for older adults: a systematic review. JAMA 2012;307:182–92.

39. Cigolle CT, Kabeto MU, Lee PG, et al. Clinical complexity and mortality in middle-aged and older adults with diabetes. J Gerontol A Biol Sci Med Sci 2012. http://dx.doi.org/10.1093/Gerona/gls095.

40. Halter JB, Merritt-Hackel J. Diabetes in the elderly population: pathophysiology, prevention, and management. Transl Endocrinol Metab 2011;2(2):9–37.

41. Ogden CL, Carroll MD. Prevalence of overweight, obesity, and extreme obesity among adults. Trends 1960-1962 through 2007-2008. United States: National Center for Health Statistics (NCHS) Health E-Stats.
42. Fakhouri TH, Ogden CL, Carroll MD, et al. Prevalence of obesity among older adults in the United States, 2007–2010. NCHS Data Brief 2012;(106):1–8.
43. Cawley J, Meyerhoefer C. The medical care costs of obesity: an instrumental variables approach. J Health Econ 2012;31(1):219. http://dx.doi.org/10.1016/j.jhealeco.2011.10.003.
44. Flegal KM, Kit BK, Orpana H, et al. Association of all-cause mortality with overweight and obesity using standard body mass index categories: a systematic review and meta-analysis. JAMA 2013;309(1):71–82.
45. Kyrou I, Tsigos C. Obesity in the elderly diabetic patient; is weight loss beneficial? No. Diabetes Care 2009;32(Supp 2):S403–13.
46. Janssen I, Mark AE. Elevated body mass index and mortality risk in the elderly. Obes Rev 2007;1:41–59.
47. Kulminiski AM, Arbeev KG, Kulminskaya IV, et al. Body mass index and nine-year mortality in disabled and nondisabled older U.S. individuals. J Am Geriatr Soc 2008;56:105–10.
48. Baumgartner RN, Stauber PM, McHugh D, et al. Cross-sectional age differences in body composition in persons 60-years of age. J Gerontol A Biol Sci Med Sci 1995;50:M307–16.
49. Manson JE, Willett WC, Stampfer MJ, et al. Body weight and mortality among women. N Engl J Med 1995;333:677–85.
50. Kuk JL, Saunders TJ, Davidson LE, et al. Age-related changes in total and regional fat distribution. Ageing Res Rev 2009;8(4):339–48.
51. Visser M, Pahor M, Tylavsky F, et al. One-and two-year change in body composition as measured by DXA in a population-based cohort of older men and women. J Appl Physiol 2003;94(6):2368–74.
52. Gallagher D, Visser M, De Meersman RE, et al. Appendicular skeletal muscle mass: effects of age, gender, and ethnicity. J Appl Physiol 1997;83:229–39.
53. Stevens J, Cai J, Pamuk ER, et al. The effect of age on the association between body-mass index and mortality. N Engl J Med 1998;338:1–7.
54. Greenberg AS, McDaniel ML. Identifying the links between obesity, insulin resistance and beta-cell function: potential role of adipocyte-derived cytokines in the pathogenesis of type 2 diabetes. Eur J Clin Invest 2001;32(Suppl 3):24–34.
55. Kahn SE, Hull RL, Utzchneider KM. Mechanisms linking obesity to insulin resistance and type 2 diabetes. Nature 2006;444:840–6.
56. Park YW, Zhu S, Palaniappan L, et al. The metabolic syndrome: prevalence and associated risk factor findings in the US population from the Third National Health and Nutrition Examination Survey, 1988–1994. Arch Intern Med 2003;163:427–36.
57. Goodpaster BH, Krishnaswami S, Harris TB, et al. Obesity, regional body fat distribution, and the metabolic syndrome in older men and women. Arch Intern Med 2005;165:777–83.
58. Andres R, Muller DC, Sorkin JD. Long-term effects of change in body weight on all-cause mortality. A review. Ann Intern Med 1993;119:737–43.
59. Williamson DF, Pamuk ER. The association between weight loss and increased longevity. A review of the evidence. Ann Intern Med 1993;119:731–6.
60. Lee IM, Paffenbarger RS Jr. Is weight loss hazardous? Nutr Rev 1996;54:S116–24.
61. Lissner L, Odell PM, D'Agostino RB, et al. Variability of body weight and health outcomes in the Framingham population. N Engl J Med 1991;324:1839–44.

62. Williamson DF, Pamuk E, Thun M, et al. Prospective study of intentional weight loss and mortality in never smoking overweight US white women aged 40–64 years. Am J Epidemiol 1995;141:1128–41.
63. Williamson DF, Pamuk E, Thun M, et al. Prospective study of intentional weight loss and mortality in overweight white men aged 40–64 years. Am J Epidemiol 1999;149:491–503.
64. Williamson DF, Thompson TJ, Thun M, et al. Intentional weight loss and mortality among overweight individuals with diabetes. Diabetes Care 2000;23:1499–504.
65. Yaari S, Goldbourt U. Voluntary and involuntary weight loss: associations with long term mortality in 9,228 middle-aged and elderly men. Am J Epidemiol 1998;148:546–55.
66. Diehr P, Bild DE, Harris TB, et al. Body mass index and mortality in nonsmoking older adults: the Cardiovascular Health Study. Am J Public Health 1998;88:623–9.
67. French SA, Folsom AR, Jeffery RW, et al. Prospective study of intentionality of weight loss and mortality in older women: the Iowa Women's Health Study. Am J Epidemiol 1999;149:504–14.
68. Wannamethee SG, Shaper AG, Lennon L. Reasons for intentional weight loss, unintentional weight loss, and mortality in older men. Arch Intern Med 2005;165:1035–40.
69. Diabetes Prevention Program Research Group. 10-year follow-up of diabetes incidence and weight loss in the diabetes prevention program outcomes study. Lancet 2009;374:1677–86.
70. Rejeski WJ, Ip EH, Bertoni AG, et al, Look AHEAD Research Group. Lifestyle change and mobility in obese adults with type 2 diabetes. N Engl J Med 2012;366:1209–21.
71. Villareal DT, Chode S, Parimi N, et al. Weight loss, exercise, or both and physical function in obese older adults. N Engl J Med 2011;364(13):1218–29.
72. Crandall J, Schade D, Ma Y, et al, Diabetes Prevention Program Research Group. The influence of age on the effects of lifestyle modification and metformin in prevention of diabetes. J Gerontol A Biol Sci Med Sci 2006;61:1075–81.
73. The Look AHEAD Research Group. Eight-year weight losses with an intensive lifestyle intervention. Obesity (Silver Spring) 2014;22(1):5–13. http://dx.doi.org/10.1002/oby.20662.
74. Varela JE, Wilson SE, Nguyen NT. Outcomes of bariatric surgery in the elderly. Am Surg 2006;72(10):865–9.
75. Sugerman HJ, DeMaria EJ, Kellum JM, et al. Effects of bariatric surgery in older patients. Ann Surg 2004;240(2):243–7.

Antidiabetic Medications and Polypharmacy

Emily P. Peron, PharmD, MS, BCPS[a],*, Kelechi C. Ogbonna, PharmD, CGP[b],
Krista L. Donohoe, PharmD, BCPS, CGP[c]

KEYWORDS

- Polypharmacy • Adverse drug events • Diabetic complications
- Hypoglycemic agents • Geriatric syndromes

KEY POINTS

- Polypharmacy, or the use of multiple medications, is common in older adults and more prevalent in older adults with diabetes.
- Medications used to treat diabetes and its complications may be associated with falls, fractures, weight changes, cognitive changes, heart disease, and urinary incontinence.
- Shared decision-making should be implemented to ensure appropriate goals of care for older adults with diabetes.

INTRODUCTION

Polypharmacy, defined as the use of multiple medications, increases with age.[1] Multiple medications are commonly prescribed for older adults, who may also contribute to complicated regimens by purchasing over-the-counter medications and dietary supplements with or without their providers' knowledge. Among community-dwelling older adults in the United States, 57% of women and 59% of men report using 5 or more medications (ie, prescription medications, over-the-counter medications, and dietary supplements) on a weekly basis. Nearly 20% report taking 10 or more medications.[1] Older adults with diabetes are at greater risk of receiving polypharmacy than those without diabetes.[2]

Achieving a balance between overprescribing, underprescribing, and appropriate prescribing can be a challenge for providers, especially those involved in the care of

[a] Geriatric Pharmacotherapy Program, Department of Pharmacotherapy & Outcomes Science, Virginia Commonwealth University, Smith Building, Room 338, 410 North 12th Street, PO Box 980533, Richmond, VA 23298-0533, USA; [b] Geriatric Pharmacotherapy Program, Department of Pharmacotherapy & Outcomes Science, Virginia Commonwealth University, Smith Building, Room 336, 410 North 12th Street, PO Box 980533, Richmond, VA 23298-0533, USA; [c] Geriatric Pharmacotherapy Program, Department of Pharmacotherapy & Outcomes Science, Virginia Commonwealth University, Smith Building, Room 220B, 410 North 12th Street, PO Box 980533, Richmond, VA 23298-0533, USA
* Corresponding author.
E-mail address: epperon@vcu.edu

Clin Geriatr Med 31 (2015) 17–27
http://dx.doi.org/10.1016/j.cger.2014.08.017   **geriatric.theclinics.com**

complex older adults. In a hypothetical 79-year-old woman with hypertension, diabetes, osteoporosis, osteoarthritis, and chronic obstructive pulmonary disease, applying clinical practice guidelines would yield 12 separate medications. Moreover, the regimen would require 19 doses per day taken at 5 different times of the day.[3] This example demonstrates the need for additional guidance beyond guideline-based care.

Although the use of multiple medications is not always inappropriate, polypharmacy is associated with increased risks of medication nonadherence,[4] drug-drug interactions,[5] and adverse drug events.[6] As such, medication reconciliation and assessments of medication adherence and potential barriers to adherence are recommended at each patient appointment.[7] The presence of polypharmacy is also associated with prescribing cascades,[8] in which adverse drug events are misinterpreted as new medical conditions and result in the prescription of new medications to treat those conditions.

FACTORS CONTRIBUTING TO POLYPHARMACY IN OLDER ADULTS WITH DIABETES

Management of hyperglycemia, microvascular complications (eg, diabetic nephropathy, neuropathy, and retinopathy) and macrovascular complications (eg, coronary artery disease, peripheral arterial disease, stroke), geriatric syndromes associated with diabetes (eg, cognitive impairment, falls, urinary incontinence), and adverse drug events contribute to an increased number of medications among older adults with diabetes. Quality improvement measures and pay-for-performance initiatives aimed at management of diabetes and its complications may improve objective measures but also contribute to the addition of unnecessary medications to the drug regimen.[3] For example, adhering to non–age-specific clinical practice guidelines for A1C goals may result in the unsafe addition of antidiabetic agents, thus leading to tighter glycemic control and increased risk of hypoglycemia and other adverse drug events. In light of recent guidance documents from the American Geriatrics Society[7] and the American Diabetes Association,[2] age- and patient-specific factors should be considered to accurately assess quality and performance.

Direct-to-consumer advertising may also contribute to polypharmacy in older adults with diabetes. In recent years, there has been a surge of new formulations of antidiabetic drugs and even new antidiabetic medication classes brought to market (**Table 1**). In some cases, these agents deliver more convenient dosing and administration and lower risks of hypoglycemia than standard alternatives, like sulfonylureas and insulin. However, early adoption of new therapies for any medical condition can be of concern in older adults, as this patient population is at increased risk of experiencing adverse drug events and may experience different adverse drug events than their younger counterparts. Moreover, as a result of direct-to-consumer advertising, patients with diabetes may seek medication therapy for diseases other than diabetes, such as erectile dysfunction or restless legs syndrome, which can further contribute to the presence of polypharmacy.

RISKS OF ANTIDIABETIC MEDICATIONS IN OLDER ADULTS

Although nonpharmacologic interventions are important in the management of diabetes, medications are a mainstay of therapy. It is particularly important when treating older adults with diabetes that the risks and benefits of pharmacologic interventions are weighed and discussed with patients and their caregivers to allow for shared decision-making. What makes treating diabetes in older adults even more complex is that the risks versus benefits for an individual are rarely clear from the clinical data available. Medications used to treat diabetes and its complications may be associated with a

Table 1
FDA-approved antidiabetic medications

Drug Class	Drug Name, Generic (Trade)
Alpha-glucosidase inhibitor	Acarbose (Precose) Miglitol (Glyset)
Amylin analog	Pramlintide (Symlin)
Biguanide	Metformin[a] (Glucophage)
Dipeptidyl peptidase-4 (DPP-4) inhibitor	Alogliptin[a] (Nesina) Linagliptin[a] (Tradjenta) Saxagliptin[a] (Onglyza) Sitagliptin[a] (Januvia)
Glucagon-like peptide-1 (GLP-1) agonist	Exenatide (Byetta) Liraglutide (Victoza) Albiglutide (Tanzeum)
Insulin	Inhalation Powder (Exubera; Afrezza) NPH[a] (Humulin N; Novolin N) Regular[a] (Humulin R; Novolin R)
Insulin analog	Aspart[a] (Novolog) Detemir (Levemir) Glargine (Lantus) Glulisine (Apidra) Lispro[a] (Humalog)
Meglitinide	Nateglinide (Starlix) Repaglinide[a] (Prandin)
Sodium-glucose co-transporter 2 (SGLT2) inhibitor	Canagliflozin (Invokana) Dapagliflozin (Farxiga) Empagliflozin (Jardiance)
Sulfonylurea – first generation	Chlorpropamide (Diabinese) Tolazamide (Tolinase) Tolbutamide (Orinase)
Sulfonylurea – second generation	Glyburide[a] (Diabeta; Glynase) Glipizide[a] (Glucotrol) Glimepiride[a] (Amaryl)
TZD	Pioglitazone[a] (Actos) Rosiglitazone[a] (Avandia)
Bile acid sequestrant	Colesevelam (Welchol)
Dopamine agonist	Bromocriptine (Cycloset)

[a] Also available in combination formulations with other antidiabetic agents.

Data from Pharmacist's letter. PL detail-document #290807. Drugs for Type 2 Diabetes. Therapeutic Research Center, August 2013; US Food and Drug Administration. FDA-approved diabetes medicines. 2013. Available at: http://www.fda.gov/ForConsumers/ByAudience/ForPatientAdvocates/DiabetesInfo/ucm294713.htm. Accessed January 5, 2014; US Food and Drug Administration. FDA news release: FDA approves Farxiga to treat type 2 diabetes. 2014. Available at: http://www.fda.gov/NewsEvents/Newsroom/PressAnnouncements/ucm380829.htm. Accessed July 15, 2014; and FDA Approved Drugs 2014. Center Watch. Available at: http://www.centerwatch.com/drug-information/fda-approved-drugs/year/2014. Accessed September 23, 2014.

host of negative outcomes that must be considered, including falls, fractures, weight changes, cognitive changes, heart disease, and urinary incontinence.

Falls

The etiology of diabetes and falls is complex and multidimensional. Peripheral neuropathy, which is present in 50% to 70% of older patients with diabetes, can increase the risk of falls and functional impairment.[7] Polypharmacy can also contribute to falls.[7] Specific antidiabetic medications that cause hypoglycemia, like insulin, have also been associated with falls.[9,10] On the other hand, untreated or undertreated hyperglycemia can also contribute to falls.[7] Antihypertensive agents, which are commonly used by patients with diabetes, have also been associated with falls[9]; however, this section will focus mainly on antidiabetic agents.

Hypoglycemia is a risk factor for falls.[9] Insulin, insulin analogs, and insulin secretagogues (ie, meglitinides and sulfonylureas) are the antidiabetic medications that predominantly cause hypoglycemia.[11] Insulin use has been shown to increase the risk of falls in older adults.[10] Insulin has a high risk of hypoglycemia; the risk of hypoglycemia may be less with insulin analogs.[11] For example, insulin glargine (Lantus) and insulin detemir (Levemir) may have a lower risk of hypoglycemia than neutral protamine Hagedorn (NPH) (Humulin N, Novolin N). Rapid-acting insulin analogs, such as lispro (Humalog), aspart (NovoLog), and glulisine (Apidra), are also associated with a lower frequency of hypoglycemia than regular insulin (Humulin R; Novolin R).[11]

Sulfonylureas have a high risk of hypoglycemia, which may be an issue for older patients. Glyburide (Diabeta; Glynase), a sulfonylurea with a long duration of action, has a greater risk of severe, prolonged hypoglycemia in older adults compared with glipizide (Glucotrol) and is a potentially inappropriate medication in this population.[12] The meglitinides are used to treat postprandial hyperglycemia. They have shorter half-lives and a lower risk of hypoglycemia than sulfonylureas.[7] Although hypoglycemia is a known risk factor for falls, there are no specific trials to date that link insulin secretagogues to falls.[13]

Dipeptidyl peptidase-4 inhibitors and glucagonlike peptide-1 agonists target postprandial hyperglycemia and impart little risk for hypoglycemia.[7] Hypoglycemia is not common with metformin (Glucophage), thiazolidinediones (TZDs), or α-glucosidase inhibitors.[11] No direct link exists between metformin and falls; however, because of metformin-induced vitamin B_{12} deficiency resulting in neuropathy, there may be an indirect association.[13] To date, there are no studies linking other antidiabetic medications to falls.[13]

Older adults with diabetes are at increased risk for injurious falls requiring hospitalization compared with those without diabetes.[10] In addition, certain risk factors, such as using insulin, a history of falls, poor standing balance score, and an A1C value $\geq 8\%$ can contribute to a fall requiring hospitalization.[10] Strategies that may help diabetic patients reduce their risk of falling include the following:

- Perform medication reviews on all prescription and over-the-counter medications to identify those that could put older adults at high risk for falls.[14]
- Limit the number of medications or doses.[14]
- Avoid hypoglycemia and hyperglycemia.[7]
- Counsel patients and caregivers on the signs and symptoms of hypoglycemia and how to manage it.[9]

Fractures

Because of the higher risk of falls associated with diabetes noted above, injurious falls resulting in fractures may occur.[10] TZDs have been shown to reduce bone mineral density and are also associated with bone fractures.[15] A longitudinal, observational cohort study in older adults showed an increased risk of fractures in those taking a TZDs compared with oral sulfonylureas or metformin.[15] Another longitudinal, observational cohort study looked to identify the time to fracture with TZDs and the risk of fracture in subgroups defined by sex and age.[16] The study suggests that in patients with diabetes, TZD use is associated with an increased risk of fractures in women, especially those older than 65 years, and after an exposure of approximately 1 year.[16] Weighing the risks versus benefits of TZD use in this population should be considered before initiating treatment.

Weight

Antidiabetic medications may cause weight loss or weight gain. As such, it may be prudent to evaluate if drug-induced weight loss may be detrimental to a patient's well-being, especially in cases of frail older adults and those experiencing unintentional weight loss. For example, in the Rancho Bernardo cohort study of 1801 community-dwelling older adults with and without diabetes, weight loss of 10 pounds or more over a 10-year period was associated with higher age-adjusted death rates over the next 12 years compared with stable weight or weight gain.[17] (See the article by Rothberg and colleagues elsewhere in this issue for a detailed discussion of weight change in older adults.)

Metformin is often considered first-line therapy in type 2 diabetes.[7] Most patients on metformin lose weight; other patients maintain weight on the drug.[18] About 88% of the weight loss associated with metformin is a result of losing body fat mass.[18] Glucagon-like peptide-1 agonists are also associated with weight loss.[7,19]

Dipeptidyl peptidase-4 inhibitors and α-glucosidase inhibitors are considered to be weight neutral.[19]

Sulfonylureas may contribute to weight gain. On initiation of sulfonylureas, many patients experience more than a 2-kg weight gain.[18] Meglitinides may also contribute to weight gain.[7] TZDs also are associated with weight gain, causing a redistribution of adipose tissue from visceral to subcutaneous depots.[18] Additionally, TZDs can cause edema, which may lead to an increase in weight. Insulin can cause significant weight gain.[7,19]

Cognition

Metformin, a biguanide, is associated with impaired cognitive performance in patients with diabetes.[20] Vitamin B_{12} deficiency in patients who take metformin is reported to be about 30%.[20] Vitamin B_{12} and calcium supplements may alleviate metformin-induced vitamin B_{12} deficiency and have been associated with better cognitive outcomes, suggesting that metformin-associated cognitive impairment is partially caused by vitamin B_{12} deficiency.[20] In older adults with diabetes who take metformin, monitoring of cognitive function is warranted.[20] Adequately powered, prospective, controlled trials are needed to explore the association between diabetes, cognitive decline, and the effect of metformin as well as the possible advantageous effects of using vitamin B_{12} or calcium supplements to help improve cognition in this population.[20] Of note, vitamin B_{12} deficiency is also a potential cause of peripheral neuropathy and should be considered in patients reporting symptoms, especially those taking metformin for long periods of time.[2]

Heart Disease

TZDs increase the risk for heart failure.[21] They may cause or exacerbate existing heart failure.[22] In patients with signs and symptoms of New York Heart Association class III or IV congestive heart failure, initiation of these agents is contraindicated.[22] After initiation or dose increases of a TZD, patients should be observed for signs and symptoms of heart failure, including excessive rapid weight gain, dyspnea, and edema.[22] If these signs or symptoms develop after heart failure is confirmed, appropriate management for heart failure should be initiated, and a discontinuation or dose reduction of the TZD should be considered.[22]

Rosiglitazone (Avandia), a TZD, has been associated with an increased risk of myocardial infarction in short-term studies; however, the US Food and Drug

Administration (FDA) determined that data for rosiglitazone-containing drugs do not show an increased risk of myocardial infarction compared with metformin and sulfo-nylureas.[23] As a result, the FDA states that distribution of the medication should no longer be restricted.[23]

Urinary Incontinence

A new antidiabetic medication class, sodium-glucose cotransporter-2 inhibitors, will need additional studies in older adults to assess if drug-associated urinary inconti-nence and urinary tract infections may be an issue in this population.[7,24]

MERGING CONCEPTS WITH PRACTICE

Managing diabetes in an older adult requires careful consideration of comorbidities, medications, and physiologic changes. In practice, providers are often faced with pacifying measures that are disease-specific or guideline-based. Older adult patients are not easily grouped by presentation, health status, or a single disease, making attainment of generalized goals more challenging.[25] A variety of guidelines exist for the management of diabetes; however, their focus on a single disease limits their application in a population with high chronic disease burden and multiple medica-tions.[3,26] To provide older adults with appropriate diabetes care, multidisciplinary strategies must be used to ensure incorporation of geriatric-based principles.

Chronologic Age Versus Physiologic Age

First and foremost, chronologic age may not equate with physiologic age. A 64-year-old patient with diabetes is very different from another 64-year-old who has diabetes in addition to heart failure, hypertension, and chronic obstructive pulmonary disease. Management in the latter patient is more complex and will likely result in the clinician and patient shifting goals of care. Although age is important, an older adult's comor-bidities and functional status should also be considered. Therefore, it is imperative that providers treat the patient rather than their specific age.

Determining life expectancy is one way in which providers can develop appropriate goals of care for an older patient with diabetes.[2,27,28] Patients with life expectancy less than 5 years are unlikely to benefit from intensive therapy, whereas those with life ex-pectancy greater than 10 years may be appropriate candidates for intensive control.[7,29] Several tools for predicting mortality have been developed and can be used as initial guides for determining intensity of therapy; however, broad application in the clinical setting is limited.[30–32] Wells and colleagues[33] developed a mortality prediction model specific to diabetes. The tool takes into account 19 different variables, including disease-related medications, blood pressure, and renal function. Although the tool was validated in a population of more than 33,000 and has a concordance index of 0.752 (correct predictability 75.2% of the time), the tool fails to take into account func-tional status and generalizability is limited to the population characteristics of the group in which it was studied.[33] The study population was predominantly white and relatively young (age range, 44–79 years) with low rates of renal impairment (31% with glomerular filtration rate < 60 mL/min), highlighting the need for more data in the oldest old (those 85 years and older) and in patient populations most affected by diabetes.

This type of prediction model can be useful as a starting point; however, the results require translation to life expectancy for an older adult. Furthermore, clinicians should be mindful of variables not captured by available tools that could easily influence dia-betes management. These variables include functional status, drug-disease interac-tions, and geriatric syndromes. Providers can estimate an older adult's approximate life expectancy compared with the median for like individuals by considering the presence or absence of unusually good or poor health and function, which will, in turn, determine trajectory of care.

Microvascular and Macrovascular Complications

The primary goal of diabetes management is to prevent and control hyperglycemia without predisposing patients to adverse events. Untreated hyperglycemia can lead to both macrovascular and microvascular complications. Before therapeutic intervention, clinicians should consider the magnitude of risk associated with each complication.

The risk of macrovascular complications, as it relates to morbidity and mortality, far exceeds the risk associated with microvascular complications in older adults with diabetes.[29] Although the United Kingdom Prospective Diabetes Study (UKPDS) excluded patients older than 65 years age at the time of enrollment, researchers observed microvascular complications in 9% of people with type 2 diabetes after 9 years of follow-up compared with rates of 20% for macrovascular complications.[29,34,35] It can be postulated that this difference between endpoints would have been even larger if more older adults were included during enrollment. Vijan and colleagues[36] evaluated the incidence of microvascular disease with increasing age and found a decline in microvascular risk as the age of type 2 diabetes onset increases (**Table 2**). In addition, the authors found the greatest improvement in microvascular complications when improving A1C value from poor to moderate (A1C 11%–9%) compared with moderate to goal (A1C 9%–7%).[37] Both studies show the importance of understanding risk associated with diabetes in the geriatric population and altering goals of care to achieve the best patient outcomes. Additional studies with emphasis on risks versus benefits of differing therapeutic goals and treatment approaches in older adults should be completed to better understand disease progression and, in turn, help guide management, drug therapy, and monitoring. Ultimately, the provider's care plan should be based on age of onset, function, life expectancy, and, most importantly, goals of care agreed on by the patient and provider.

Macrovascular complications, such as coronary artery disease and stroke, pose the greatest risk to older adults with diabetes. There are 10.9 million Americans 65 years or older with diabetes, representing nearly 30% of this population segment. In the US, diabetes is the seventh leading cause of mortality with 69,071 deaths in 2010 alone. Among people 64 years or older, cardiovascular disease accounts for 68% of diabetes-related deaths.[38]

Table 2
Lifetime Risk of End-Stage Renal Disease (%)/Lifetime Risk of Blindness from Diabetic Retinopathy (%)

Hemoglobin A$_{1c}$ Level	Age at Onset of Diabetes			
	45 y	55 y	65 y	75 y
7	2.0/0.3	0.9/0.1	0.3/<0.1	0.1/<0.1
8	2.7/1.1	1.3/0.5	0.5/0.2	0.1/<0.1
9	3.5/2.6	1.6/1.2	0.6/0.5	0.1/0.1
10	4.3/5.0	2.1/2.5	0.8/1.0	0.2/0.3
11	5.0/7.9	2.5/4.4	0.9/1.9	2.2/0.5

Data from Vijan S, Hofer TP, Hayward RA. Estimated benefits of glycemic control in microvascular complications in type 2 diabetes. Ann Intern Med 1997;127(9):788–95. http://dx.doi.org/10.7326/0003-4819-127-9-199711010-00003.

To understand the role of glycemic intervention on cardiovascular endpoints 3 pivotal randomized, control trials (the Action to Control Cardiovascular Risk in Diabetes [ACCORD] trial, the Action in Diabetes and Vascular Disease: Preterax and Diamicron MR Controlled Evaluation [ADVANCE] trial, and the Veterans Affairs Diabetes Trial [VADT]) were completed. All 3 trials incorporated an intensive therapy arm with a goal A1C value of less than 6.0% or less than 6.5%. The ACCORD trial ended early (after 3 years) because of excessive deaths in the intensive glucose control arm.[38,39] Post-hoc analysis of the VADT trial also suggests that mortality risk increases with increasing duration of diabetes. Those with diabetes for less than 15 years received benefit, whereas those with diabetes for 20 years or more had a higher mortality rate in the intensive therapy arm.[40,41] To the contrary, the ADVANCE trial did not observe an increased risk of mortality in the intensive glucose control arm over a median follow-up of 5 years.[42]

Although the results for 2 of the 3 trials favor more lenient glycemic control for older adults with diabetes, uncertainty remains. Treating older adults with diabetes requires deliberate and thoughtful interventions. More studies focusing on the oldest old must be conducted to challenge our assumptions, particularly as we prepare to care for an increasingly aged population. Until more data are available, clinicians must weigh the potential risks of therapy with the potential benefits of reducing the excess morbidity and mortality associated with diabetes.

PATIENT-CENTERED CARE AND QUALITY OF LIFE

Given the intricacy and variability of diabetes management in the geriatric population, patient involvement and shared decision-making are essential. Positive outcomes in this patient population rely heavily on the patient's or caregiver's ability to manage multiple chronic diseases and medications on a daily basis. Patient-centered care is defined as an approach to "providing care that is respectful of and responsive to individual preferences, needs, and values and ensuring the patient values guide all clinical decisions."[43,44] Clinicians should actively engage patients in clinical decisions by helping patients prioritize treatment options consistent with their goals and preferences while also accounting for the magnitude and time to benefit in the context of the patient's overall health.[45] Often when this shared decision-making model is implemented, providers are given a greater perspective on patient's needs and ability to manage their diabetes in the setting of other chronic conditions. Ultimately, it is the patient's decision to implement or forgo therapy based on their needs and wishes to maintain their own definition of quality of life.

SUMMARY

Polypharmacy, or the use of multiple medications, is a common concern in older adults with diabetes. Age, comorbidities, and microvascular and macrovascular complications of diabetes may further complicate diabetes management in older adults. Moreover, older adults may be more sensitive to potentially serious adverse effects of antidiabetic medications, including cognitive changes. Diabetic care in the elderly should not focus on any one of these aspects alone; instead, a comprehensive approach should be used with the patient's goals of care in mind.

REFERENCES

1. Slone Epidemiology Center. Patterns of medication use in the United States. Available at: http://www.bu.edu/slone/files/2012/11/SloneSurveyReport2006.pdf. 2006. Accessed January 25, 2014.

2. American Diabetes Association. Standards of medical care in diabetes – 2014. Diabetes Care 2014;37(Suppl.1):S14–80. http://dx.doi.org/10.2337/dc14-S014.
3. Boyd CM, Darer J, Boult C, et al. Clinical practice guidelines and quality of care for older patients with multiple comorbid diseases: implications for pay for performance. JAMA 2005;294(6):716–24. http://dx.doi.org/10.1001/jama.294.6.716.
4. Murray MD, Darnell J, Weinberger M, et al. Factors contributing to medication noncompliance in elderly public housing tenants. Drug Intell Clin Pharm 1986; 20(2):146–52.
5. Ferner RE, Aronson JK. Communicating information about drug safety. BMJ 2006;333(7559):143–5. http://dx.doi.org/10.1136/bmj.333.7559.143.
6. Field TS, Gurwitz JH, Avorn J, et al. Risk factors for adverse drug events among nursing home residents. Arch Intern Med 2001;161(31):1629–34. http://dx.doi.org/10.1001/archinte.161.13.1629.
7. Kirkman MS, Briscoe VJ, Clark N, et al. Diabetes in older adults: a consensus report. J Am Geriatr Soc 2012;60(12):2342–56. http://dx.doi.org/10.1111/jgs.12035.
8. Rochon PA, Gurwitz JH. Optimising drug treatment for elderly people: the prescribing cascade. BMJ 1997;314(7115):1096–9. http://dx.doi.org/10.1136/bmj.315.7115.1096.
9. Keller RB, Slattum PW. Strategies for prevention of medication-related falls in the elderly. Consult Pharm 2003;18(3):248–58.
10. Yau RK, Strotmeyer ES, Resnick HE, et al. Diabetes and risk of hospitalized injury among older adults. Diabetes Care 2013;36(12):3985–91. http://dx.doi.org/10.2337/dc13-0429.
11. Zammitt NN, Frier BM. Hypoglycemia in type 2 diabetes: pathophysiology, frequency, and effects of different treatment modalities. Diabetes Care 2005; 28(12):2948–61. http://dx.doi.org/10.2337/diacare.28.12.2948.
12. American Geriatrics Society. 2012 Beers Criteria Update Expert Panel. American Geriatrics Society updated Beers criteria for potentially inappropriate medication use in older adults. J Am Geriatr Soc 2012;60(4):616–31. http://dx.doi.org/10.1111/j.1532-5415.2012.03923.x.
13. Berlie HD, Garwood CL. Diabetes medications related to an increased risk of falls and fall-related morbidity in the elderly. Ann Pharmacother 2010;44(4):712–7. http://dx.doi.org/10.1345/aph.1M551.
14. The American Geriatrics Society. 2010 AGS/BGS clinical practice guideline: prevention of falls in older persons. Available at: http://www.american-geriatrics.org/health_care_professionals/clinical_practice/clinical_guidelines_ recommendations/2010/. Accessed January 5, 2013.
15. Solomon DH, Cadarette SM, Choudhry NK, et al. A cohort study of thiazolidinediones and fractures in older adults with diabetes. J Clin Endocrinol Metab 2009;94(8):2792–8. http://dx.doi.org/10.1210/jc.2008-2157.
16. Zeina HA, Havstad SL, Wells K, et al. Thiazolidinedione use and the longitudinal risk of fractures in patients with type 2 diabetes mellitus. J Clin Endocrinol Metab 2010;95(2):592–600. http://dx.doi.org/10.1210/jc.2009-1385.
17. Wedick NM, Barrett-Connor E, Knoke JD, et al. The relationship between weight loss and all-cause mortality in older men and women with and without diabetes mellitus: the Rancho Bernardo study. J Am Geriatr Soc 2002;50(11):1810–5.
18. Fowler MJ. Diabetes treatment, part 2: oral agents for glycemic management. Clin Diabetes 2007;25(4):131–4. http://dx.doi.org/10.2337/diaclin.25.4.131.
19. Hermansen K, Mortensen LS. Bodyweight changes associated with antihyperglycaemic agents in type 2 diabetes mellitus. Drug Saf 2007;30(12):1127–42. http://dx.doi.org/10.2165/00002018-200730120-00005.

20. Moore EM, Mander AG, Ames D, et al. Increased risk of cognitive impairment in patients with diabetes is associated with metformin. Diabetes Care 2013;36(10): 2981–7. http://dx.doi.org/10.2337/dc13-0229.

21. Singh S, Loke YK, Furberg CD. Thiazolidinediones and heart failure: a teleo-analysis. Diabetes Care 2007;30(8):2148–53. http://dx.doi.org/10.2337/dc07-0141.

22. U.S. Food and Drug Administration. Information for healthcare professionals: Pio-glitazone HCl (marketed as Actos, Actoplus Met, and Duetact). Published August 2007. Updated August 14, 2013. Available at: http://www.fda.gov/Drugs/DrugSafety/PostmarketDrugSafetyInformationforPatientsandProviders/ucm124178.htm. Accessed January 5, 2014.

23. U.S. Food and Drug Administration. FDA Drug Safety Communication: FDA re-quires removal of some prescribing and dispensing restrictions for rosiglitazone-containing diabetes medicines. Published November 29, 2013. Updated January 9, 2014. Available at: http://www.fda.gov/Drugs/DrugSafety/ucm376389.htm. Ac-cessed February 15, 2014.

24. Invokana (canagliflozin) [package insert]. Titusville (NJ): Janssen Pharmaceuti-cals, Inc; 2013.

25. Boyd CM, McNabney MK, Brandt N, et al. Guiding principles for the care of older adults with multimorbidity: an approach for clinicians. J Am Geriatr Soc 2012; 60(10):E1–25. http://dx.doi.org/10.1111/j.1532-5415.2012.04188.x.

26. Tinetti ME, Bogardus ST Jr, Agostini JV. Potential pitfalls of disease-specific guidelines for patients with multiple conditions. N Engl J Med 2004;351(27): 2870–4. http://dx.doi.org/10.1056/NEJMsb042458.

27. Brown AF, Mangione CM, Saliba D, et al. Guidelines for improving the care of the older person with diabetes mellitus. J Am Geriatr Soc 2003;51(5 Suppl Guidelines):S265–80. http://dx.doi.org/10.1046/j.1532-5415.51.5s.1.x.

28. Sinclair AJ, Paolisso G, Castro M, et al. European Diabetes Working Party for older people 2011 clinical guidelines for type 2 diabetes mellitus. Executive sum-mary. Diabetes Metab 2011;37(Suppl. 3):S27–38. http://dx.doi.org/10.1016/S1262-3636(11)70962-4.

29. Wallace JI. Management of diabetes in the elderly. Clin Diabetes 1999;17(1): 19–25. Available at: http://journal.diabetes.org/clinicaldiabetes/v17n11999/Pg19.htm. Accessed February 15, 2014.

30. Yourman LC, Lee SJ, Schonberg MA, et al. Prognostic indices for older adults: a systematic review. JAMA 2012;307(2):182–92. http://dx.doi.org/10.1001/jama.2011.1966.

31. Lee SJ, Lindquist K, Segal MR, et al. Development and validation of a prognostic index for 4-year mortality in older adults. JAMA 2006;295(7):801–8. http://dx.doi.org/10.1001/jama.295.7.801.

32. Schonberg MA, Davis RB, McCarthy EP, et al. Index to predict 5-year mortality of community-dwelling adults aged 65 and older using data from the National Health Interview Survey. J Gen Intern Med 2009;24(10):1115–22. http://dx.doi.org/10.1007/s11606-009-1073-y.

33. Wells BJ, Jain A, Arrigain S, et al. Predicting 6-year mortality risk in patients with type 2 diabetes. Diabetes Care 2008;31(12):2301–6. http://dx.doi.org/10.2337/dc08-1047.

34. UK Prospective Diabetes Study (UKPDS) Group. Effect of intensive blood-glucose control with metformin on complications in overweight patients with type 2 diabetes (UKPDS 34). Lancet 1998;352(9139):854–65. http://dx.doi.org/10.1016/S0140-6736(98)07037-8.

35. UK Prospective Diabetes Study (UKPDS) Group. Intensive blood-glucose control with sulphonylureas or insulin compared with conventional treatment and risk of complications in patients with type 2 diabetes (UKPDS 33). Lancet 1998; 352(9178):837–53. http://dx.doi.org/10.1016/S0140-6736(98)07019-6.
36. Vijan S, Hofer TP, Hayward RA. Estimated benefits of glycemic control in micro-vascular complications in type 2 diabetes. Ann Intern Med 1997;127(9): 788–95. http://dx.doi.org/10.7326/0003-4819-127-9-199711010-00003.
37. National Diabetes Education Program. The Facts about diabetes: a leading cause of death in the U.S. National Diabetes Education Program. 2007. Available at: http://ndep.nih.gov/diabetes-facts/. Accessed February 15, 2014.
38. Gerstein HC, Miller ME, Byington RP, et al. Effects of intensive glucose lowering in type 2 diabetes. N Engl J Med 2008;358(24):2545–59. http://dx.doi.org/10.1056/NEJMoa080274.
39. Miller ME, Bonds DE, Gerstein HC, et al. The effects of baseline characteristics, glycaemia treatment approach, and glycated haemoglobin concentration on the risk of severe hypoglycaemia: post hoc epidemiological analysis of the ACCORD study. BMJ 2010;340:b5444. http://dx.doi.org/10.1136/bmj.b5444.
40. Duckworth WC, Abraira C, Moritz TE, et al. Glucose control and vascular compli-cations in veterans with type 2 diabetes. N Engl J Med 2009;360(2):129–39. http://dx.doi.org/10.1056/NEJMoa0808431.
41. Duckworth WC, Abraira C, Moritz TE, et al. The duration of diabetes affects the response to intensive glucose control in type 2 subjects: the VA diabetes trial. J Diabetes Complications 2011;25(6):355–61. http://dx.doi.org/10.1016/j.jdiacomp.2011.10.003.
42. ADVANCE Collaborative Group, Patel A, MacMahon S, Chalmers J, et al. Inten-sive blood glucose control and vascular outcomes in patients with type 2 diabetes. N Engl J Med 2008;358(24):2560–72. http://dx.doi.org/10.1056/NEJMoa0802987.
43. Committee on Quality of Health Care in America: Institute of Medicine. Crossing the quality chasm: a new health system for the 21st century. Washington, DC: The National Academies Press; 2001.
44. Inzucchi SE, Bergenstal RM, Buse JB, et al. Management of hyperglycemia in type 2 diabetes: a patient-centered approach: position statement of the American Diabetes Association (ADA) and the European Association for the Study of Dia-betes (EASD). Diabetes Care 2012;35(6):1364–79. http://dx.doi.org/10.2337/dc12-0413.
45. Durso S. Using clinical guidelines designed for older adults with diabetes mellitus and complex health status. JAMA 2006;295(16):1935–40. http://dx.doi.org/10.1001/jama.295.16.1935.

Atherosclerotic Cardiovascular Disease in Older Adults with Diabetes Mellitus

Joshua I. Barzilay, MD[a,b,]*, Kenneth J. Mukamal, MD, MPH[c], Jorge R. Kizer, MD, MSc[d,e]

KEYWORDS

- Diabetes • Subclinical vascular disease • Risk • Cardiovascular disease • Mortality
- Older age

KEY POINTS

- Diabetes is a significant risk factor for cardiovascular disease and mortality into old age.
- The main manifestation of diabetes in old age is microvascular brain disease found on brain MRI.
- Newly discovered diabetes poses an immediate risk for cardiovascular disease and mortality.

INTRODUCTION

In this review article we focus on 4 specific questions relevant to the practicing physician regarding the impact of diabetes mellitus (DM) on the risk of atherosclerotic cardiovascular disease (CVD) in older adults:

1. Is DM a significant risk factor for total and CVD mortality in older people? Does diabetes have the same strength of association with total and atherosclerotic

Funding Support: This work was funded in part by R01 HL094555 from the National Heart, Lung, and Blood Institute (to K.J. Mukamal, MD, MPH, and J.R. Kizer, MD, MSc). None of the authors has a conflict of interest regarding the contents of this article.

[a] Kaiser Permanente, 3650 Steve Reynolds Boulevard, Duluth, GA 30096, USA; [b] Division of Endocrinology, Emory University School of Medicine, 101 Woodruff Circle, Suite 1303, Atlanta, GA 30322, USA; [c] Department of Medicine, Beth Israel Deaconess Medical Center, Harvard University, 330 Brookline Avenue, Boston, MA 02215, USA; [d] Department of Medicine, Albert Einstein College of Medicine, Jack and Pearl Resnick Campus, 1300 Morris Park Avenue Block, Room 114, Bronx, NY 10461, USA; [e] Department of Epidemiology and Population Health, Albert Einstein College of Medicine, Jack and Pearl Resnick Campus, 1300 Morris Park Avenue Block, Room 114, Bronx, NY 10461, USA
* Corresponding author. 3650 Steve Reynolds Boulevard, Duluth, GA 30096.
E-mail address: Joshua.barzilay@kp.org

CVD mortality in people 75 years or older as it does in younger people? Is diabetes a coronary heart disease (CHD) equivalent in older age?

2. What impact does newly discovered DM have on CVD risk?
3. What are the prime risk factors for CVD in older adults with diabetes?
4. How common is subclinical cerebrovascular disease in older adults with diabetes?

The data for this review draws primarily from our work with the Cardiovascular Health Study (CHS), an ongoing observational study of cardiovascular risk factors in adults age 65 years of age and older. CHS enrolled nearly 6000 older adults in 4 field centers across the United States between 1989 and 1993 and has followed them continuously for the occurrence of cardiovascular events, including myocardial infarction and stroke. Of particular interest, CHS administered a 2-hour oral glucose tolerance test at the initial examination for the first 5201 participants, offering the unique opportunity to address fasting and post load glucose values as risk factors for atherosclerotic vascular disease. In addition, we also review studies of other older population cohorts.

ARE MORTALITY AND ATHEROSCLEROTIC CARDIOVASCULAR DISEASE INCREASED IN OLDER ADULTS WITH DIABETES MELLITUS?

It may be argued that the impact of DM as a risk factor for vascular disease wanes with advancing age, just as happens with some traditional CVD risk factors, such as hypercholesterolemia.[1] The "wear and tear" of growing old and the high prevalence of subclinical vascular disease might attenuate the effect of DM on total and CVD mortality risk.

To examine this issue, we performed an analysis of the CHS data set from 1989 to 2001.[2] Similar to other population-based diabetes studies,[3] we adjusted for traditional risk factors such as age, sex, hypertension, and smoking status. We also included other "nontraditional" factors associated with DM. These included low levels of attained education, high rates of disability, depression, frailty, subclinical CVD, and elevated levels of inflammation factors. We found that the adjusted relative risk of total mortality for participants treated with oral hypoglycemic agents and insulin, relative to those without diabetes, was 1.33 (95% CI, 1.10–1.62) and 2.04 (95% CI, 1.62–2.57), respectively. The total mortality risk estimate for oral hypoglycemic agent users was somewhat lower than that of prior studies, whereas the estimate for insulin users was in line with prior studies.[4] For CVD mortality, the adjusted relative risks were 1.99 (95% CI, 1.54–2.57) and 2.16 (95% CI, 1.54–3.03), and for CHD estimates were 2.47 (95% CI, 1.89–3.24) and 2.75 (95% CI, 1.95–3.87), respectively. These estimates were similar to those from studies of diabetes from predominantly middle-aged cohorts from prior decades,[4] which adjusted only for traditional CVD risk factors. From these results we conclude that diabetes continues to confer a substantial increase in risk of total and CVD mortality into older age, and the addition of nontraditional risk factors does not modify these relationships in a meaningful manner (Fig. 1).

Next, we examined the effect of age on mortality risk. We included an interaction term in our models (65–74 vs >74 years of age). The term was not significant, suggesting that the effect of diabetes on total and CVD mortality outcomes between those with and without diabetes was the same whether one was less than or greater than 74 years of age. A similar conclusion was reached in an analysis of a Medicare claims dataset, which demonstrated excess mortality risk from diabetes in all age groups, including the elderly.[5] This issue is of clinical importance because there is a tendency to be less "aggressive" in risk factor management the older the patient. In contrast with our findings, the Emerging Risk Factor

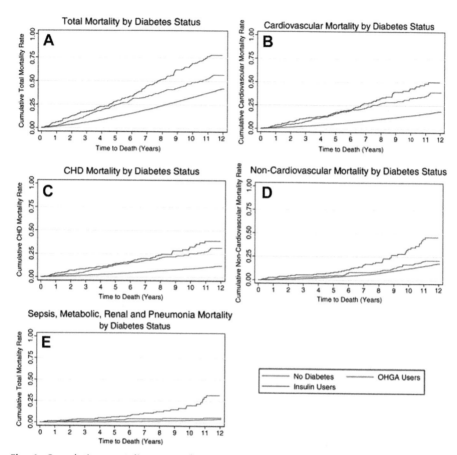

Fig. 1. Cumulative mortality curves for Cardiovascular Health Study participants with or without diabetes. Those with diabetes are further categorized as oral hypoglycemic agent users (OHGA) and insulin users. (A) Total mortality by diabetes status. (B) Cardiovascular mortality by diabetes status. (C) Coronary heart disease (CHD) mortality by diabetes status. (D) Noncardiovascular mortality by diabetes status. (E) Sepsis, metabolic, renal, and pneumonia mortality by diabetes status. (*From* Kronmal RA, Barzilay JI, Smith NL, et al. Mortality in pharmacologically treated older adults with diabetes: the Cardiovascular Health Study, 1989–2001. PLoS Med 2006;3(10):e400.)

Collaboration reported, in a meta-analysis of 102 trials with individual data on people with diabetes, that the risks of CHD and stroke events, including mortality, were lower in people with diabetes versus people without diabetes in those older than 70 years of age compared with those 60 to 69 and 40 to 59 years of age.[6] Taken together, available evidence indicates significantly increased risks of mortality and atherosclerotic CVD among elders with diabetes, although the heightened incidence of these outcomes seems less pronounced than in middle-aged cohorts.

Finally, we examined the impact of gender on total and CVD mortality in older adults with diabetes. In middle-aged cohort studies, women exhibit a higher relative risk of CVD (especially CHD) mortality compared with men.[7] In CHS, we observed a similar finding.[2] Women with diabetes had a relative total mortality risk of 2.28 (95% CI,

1.90–2.72) compared with nondiabetic women, whereas diabetic men had a relative risk of 1.80 (95% CI, 1.53–2.11). When this risk was categorized by treatment type an interesting finding emerged. Women treated with oral hypoglycemic agents had a total mortality risk similar to that of men (hazard ratio [HR], 1.62 [95% CI, 1.33–2.09] vs HR 1.63 [95% CI, 1.33–2.00], respectively). On the other hand, the relative mortality risk associated with insulin therapy was much higher in women than men (approximately 3 times higher among women compared with approximately 50% higher among men). The increased relative risk with insulin therapy for women with DM was owing mainly to the lower risk of death in women without diabetes, because women and men with diabetes treated with insulin had similarly high absolute cumulative mortality (>75% at 12-year follow-up). Thus, the loss of the mortality advantage that women have over men in the setting of diabetes is driven mainly in those who use insulin. It is in this group of women that extra diligence in management is called for.

NEWLY DIAGNOSED DIABETES: WHAT IS THE MORTALITY RISK?

Clinicians who treat older adults often come across the situation where an older person's blood glucose is elevated on a routine physical examination. The patient feels well and has no history of CVD. The question arises whether newly diagnosed diabetes poses a risk of near-term CVD. Should the physician be aggressive in managing the risk factors associated with diabetes in this older person? It may be argued that the effects of elevated glucose levels take many years to result in clinical atherosclerosis, so urgency is not necessary.

Using data from the CHS,[8] we found that new-onset diabetes, defined by the initiation of antidiabetes medication or by a fasting plasma glucose of greater than 125 mg/dL, was associated with a 90% increase in risk of all-cause mortality and a 120% increase in risk of cardiovascular mortality compared with study participants without diabetes. There was a large increase in cardiovascular mortality in the first 2 years of follow-up that diminished over time, whereas all-cause mortality risk remained consistently elevated throughout the 8 years of follow-up. There are 2 explanations for this short-term excess mortality risk. First, the limited duration of exposure to hyperglycemia may reflect more sustained exposure to associated oxidative stress, inflammation, and nonglycemic atherosclerosis risk factors (eg, hyperinsulinemia, dyslipidemia, hypertension), which increase susceptibility to atherothrombotic events. Second, newly elevated fasting glucose levels in the diabetic range reflect prolonged glucose exposure to nondiabetic hyperglycemia, which increases risk as well. Whatever is the explanation of our finding, it is important to know that newly diagnosed diabetes poses a serious and near-term risk to the elderly person.

IS DIABETES A "CARDIOVASCULAR DISEASE EQUIVALENT" IN OLDER ADULTS?

In the late 1990s, Haffner and colleagues[9] reported that diabetic patients without previous myocardial infarction had as high a risk of myocardial infarction as nondiabetic patients with previous myocardial infarction. The cohort for this study was approximately 58 years of age. Do the same findings hold true into older age? We examined the CHS dataset after a mean of 12 years follow-up and asked whether cardiovascular and all-cause mortality rates were similar between participants with prevalent CHD (confirmed history of myocardial infarction, angina, or coronary revascularization) versus participants with diabetes only.[10] We found that CHD mortality risk was virtually identical between participants with CHD alone versus diabetes alone (HR, 1.04; 95% CI, 0.83–1.30). The proportion of mortality attributable to prevalent diabetes (population-attributable risk percent 8.4%) and prevalent CHD

(6.7%) were similar in women. On the other hand, the proportion of mortality attributable to atherosclerotic heart disease (16.5%) compared with diabetes (6.4%) was higher in men. Similar patterns were found for CVD mortality. Notably, however, the adjusted hazard ratio for total mortality was significantly lower among participants with atherosclerotic heart disease alone (HR, 0.85; 95% CI, 0.75–0.96) compared with participants with DM alone.

In contrast with these data, the British Regional Heart Study (BRHS) arrived at different conclusions.[11] In the BRHS, the risk of CVD outcomes was compared among participants with (1) early diagnosis (age <60 years) and longer duration (mean, 16.7 years) of diabetes; (2) those with late diagnosis (age ≥60 years) and shorter duration (mean, 1.9 years) of diabetes; (3) those with a myocardial infarction but no diabetes; and (4) individuals without either condition (the reference group). The researchers found that risks of major CHD events and mortality were increased in participants with late onset diabetes (relative risk [RR], 1.54 [95% CI, 1.07–2.21] but less than in those with early onset diabetes (RR, 2.39 [95% CI, 1.41–4.05]) and those with prior myocardial infarction (RR, 2.51 [95% CI, 1.88–3.36]). In other words, both early and late onset of diabetes were associated with increased risk of major CHD events and mortality, but only early onset of diabetes (with >10 years' duration) seems to be a CHD equivalent. Differences in study characteristics (CHS participants were 5 years older than BRHS participants; the BRHS included only men, whereas CHS had both men and women) may account for these discordant findings.

With regard to the risk of CVD and mortality, the physician may ask what is the likelihood of a recurrent event. In a national study of diabetic patients from Italy, mean age 68 years, 6.1% of the patients with a prior CVD event developed a new major atherosclerotic complication annually, including mortality.[12] A higher rate of 7.6% per year was reported in the Drugs and Evidence-Based Medicine in the Elderly (DEBATE) study,[13] in subjects with a mean age of 80 years.

RISK FACTORS FOR ATHEROSCLEROTIC CARDIOVASCULAR DISEASE IN THE ELDERLY
Subclinical Cardiovascular Disease in Older Adults with Diabetes

The relative importance of traditional CVD risk factors tends to wane with advancing age.[14] What then is the main determinant of CVD in older diabetic adults? To answer this question, we analyzed the CHS dataset[15] after a mean follow-up of 6.4 years, adjusting for traditional CVD risk factors, as well as for the presence of subclinical CVD. The 2 risk factors that were consistently associated with CVD outcomes were age and the presence of subclinical CVD. The latter increased the risk of clinical outcomes by approximately 2-fold. The increase in risk of clinical CVD in the diabetic population of CHS was largely confined to those with prevalent subclinical CVD at baseline. The risk for the combination of diabetes and subclinical disease was more than 2-fold (HR, 2.5; 95% CI, 1.9–3.4), whereas that for diabetes with no subclinical disease was not significantly increased (HR, 1.3; 95% CI, 0.8–2.0), compared with participants with neither diabetes nor subclinical disease (**Fig. 2**). Of note, participants with impaired glucose tolerance (defined as a 2-hour glucose between 140 and 199 mg/dL), a condition that is associated with a high risk of subsequent diabetes, generally had an intermediate risk.

We have previously demonstrated that elevated low-density lipoprotein cholesterol, lower high-density lipoprotein cholesterol, and elevated triglyceride levels, along with cigarette smoking and elevated systolic blood pressure, are related to subclinical CVD.[16] Our findings suggest that once subclinical CVD has developed, these risk factors (and especially lipid levels) may have little association with clinical disease.

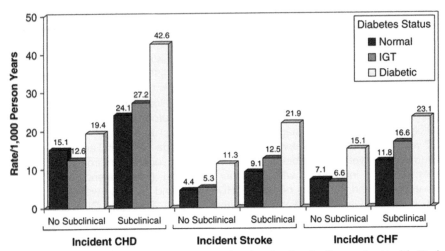

Fig. 2. Incidence of several cardiovascular end points in the Cardiovascular Health Study according to glucose status on a 2-hour oral glucose tolerance test (normal glycemia, impaired glucose tolerance [IGT], diabetes) categorized by the presence or absence of subclinical vascular disease. CHD, coronary heart disease; CHF, congestive heart failure. (*From* Kuller LH, Velentgas P, Barzilay J, et al. Diabetes mellitus: subclinical cardiovascular disease and risk of incident cardiovascular disease and all-cause mortality. Arterioscler Thromb Vasc Biol 2000;20:823–9; with permission.)

However, modifications of these risk factors may still reduce the risk of clinical disease earlier in life by modifying the extent or characteristics of subclinical disease and particularly of plaque stability and susceptibility to thrombosis.[17]

Distribution of Subclinical and Clinical Cardiovascular Disease in Older Adults with Diabetes

To clarify what subclinical CVD consists of and to better characterize the overall prevalence of CVD in older adults, we summarized the results of several complementary vascular tests that were conducted in the CHS.[18] These tests included an echocardiogram (for left ventricular hypertrophy, wall motion abnormalities, low ejection fraction), electrocardiography (for major ST and T wave changes), carotid ultrasound (for intimal medial thickness and plaque), cranial magnetic resonance imaging (for strokes and lacunar infarcts), and peripheral blood pressure measurement (for ankle arm index). Clinical disease consisted of previous myocardial infarction, coronary revascularization, angina, heart failure, stroke, and claudication. We further categorized the cohort as having normal glucose tolerance, impaired fasting glucose, newly diagnosed DM, or known DM. Impaired fasting glucose, defined as a fasting glucose of 100 to 125 mg/dL, is associated with an increased risk of subsequent diabetes.

We found that approximately 30% of the cohort had clinical CVD of at least 1 form (**Fig. 3**). The most common form was CHD. Of those without clinical disease, approximately 60% had some form of isolated subclinical disease. The most common form of such isolated subclinical disease was cerebrovascular disease. The prevalence of either clinical or isolated subclinical CVD increased with severity of the glucose disorder. The increased risk was more pronounced in women than in men, as we previously noted. Last, clinical CVD comprised a greater proportion of the total CVD burden among those with glucose disorders than among those with normal fasting glucose status (ie, CVD was relatively more likely to be clinical than subclinical in those with

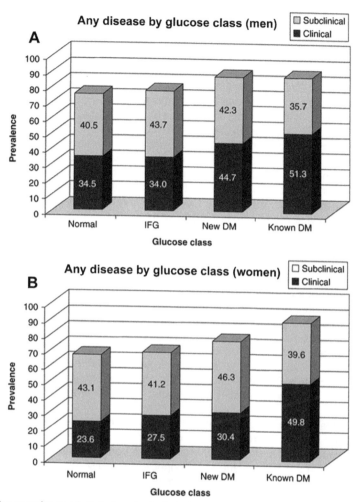

Fig. 3. The prevalence of clinical and subclinical cardiovascular disease among participants from the Cardiovascular Health Study according to glucose status on a 2-hour oral glucose tolerance test (normal glycemia, impaired glucose tolerance [IGT], diabetes [DM]). (*A*) Any disease by glucose class (men). (*B*) Any disease by glucose class (women). IFG, impaired fasting glucose. (*From* Barzilay JI, Spiekerman CF, Kuller LH, et al. Prevalence of clinical and isolated subclinical cardiovascular disease in older adults with glucose disorders. The Cardiovascular Health Study. Diabetes Care 2001;24:1233–9.)

abnormal glucose regulation). Taken together, these results support the hypothesis that glucose disorders (and associated pathophysiologic processes and metabolic changes) promote atherosclerosis and its progression from subclinical to clinical disease.

Fasting Versus Post Prandial Hyperglycemia

Aging tends to have a stronger effect on post prandial than on fasting glucose levels.[19] Given this fact, one might wonder if post prandial glucose is as strong a risk factor for CVD and mortality as fasting glucose in older adults. Our work suggests that it is strongly related to risk.[20] When we compared the American Diabetes Association criteria for diabetes based on fasting glucose levels with World Health Organization criteria that incorporate oral glucose tolerance testing (and 2-hour glucose levels), the number of cases of CVD attributable to abnormal fasting glucose states was one third that attributable to abnormal glucose tolerance. The sensitivity of fasting criteria for incident CVD was only 28%, compared with 54% using World Health Organization criteria. In similar analyses that simultaneously evaluated fasting and 2-hour glucose among CHS participants who were not receiving hypoglycemic treatment, only 2-hour glucose level was associated with risk of CVD.[21]

These findings are consistent with those reported from the Rancho Bernardo Study,[22] where isolated post prandial hyperglycemia was associated with increased risks of CHD and CVD mortality in older women, but not men. They are also compatible with the findings of the DECODE study, which likewise reported that 2-hour glucose was associated with incident CVD and mortality independent of fasting glucose, but not vice versa, across cohorts spanning the adult age range.[23]

CEREBROVASCULAR DISEASE

Diabetes is a risk factor for clinical stroke. Population-based registries of stroke report a prevalence of DM ranging from 9.5% to 20%.[24] In addition, 16% to 24% of nondiabetic patients at the time of admission for acute stroke have DM according to an oral glucose tolerance test performed 12 weeks after the stroke.[25] In the Framingham Heart Study, the proportion of CVD, including stroke, attributable to diabetes increased from 5.4% to 8.7% between 1952 and 1998.[26] In CHS,[15] we found that the risk of stroke mortality in people with diabetes was 4.1 (95% CI, 2.6–6.7) and 2.5 (95% CI, 1.3–4.8) times higher than that of nondiabetic participants depending on whether subclinical vascular disease was present or not, respectively.

Aside from large vessel cerebrovascular disease, it is now recognized that small vessel disease of the brain is much more common than large vessel disease. Computed tomography and MRI have made it apparent that a majority of cases of cerebral infarction are "silent" and not recognized clinically. Reports conflict about whether DM is a risk factor for these silent strokes. In CHS,[27] 3660 participants underwent brain MRI. Of these subjects, 2529 (69%) were free of infarcts of any kind. Another 841 (23%) had 1 or more lacunar infarcts without other stroke types present. For most of the 841 subjects, the lacunar infarcts were single (66%) and silent (89%), that is, without a history of transient ischemic attack or stroke. In multivariate analyses, people with DM had a nearly 33% higher prevalence of lacunae than people without DM. In a follow-up study[28] of 1433 CHS participants who underwent 2 MRIs separated by 5 years and who had no infarcts on the initial MRI, 254 participants (17.7%) had 1 or more infarcts. DM was not associated with these incident MRI-defined infarcts late in life. In the Rotterdam Scan Study,[29] a population-based cohort study of 1077 participants 60 to 90 years of age, participants also underwent cerebral MRI. For 259 participants (24%), 1 or more infarcts on MRI were seen; 217 persons had only silent and 42 had symptomatic infarcts. Diabetes was not related to silent strokes in this study.

A recent report may explain why there is inconsistency regarding diabetes as a risk factor for lacunar infarcts. Theories pertaining to the etiology of small brain infarcts have varied but 2 possible mechanisms have been emphasized: (1) development of microatheroma obstructing flow of small penetrating arteries and (2) the occurrence of fibrinoid necrosis in these penetrating arteries. Using data from the Atherosclerosis

Risk in Communities (ARIC) study,[30] investigators studied which risk factors were associated with infarctlike lesions of less than 20 mm in maximum dimension. Infarctlike lesions that were 7 mm or smaller in diameter were hypothesized to be owing to lipohyalinosis. Those that were 8 to 20 mm were hypothesized to reflect microatheromatous disease. If their hypothesis was correct, different risk factors associated with each size of lesion would be expected. The authors found that very small lesions were associated with diabetes or elevated hemoglobin A1c levels. Metabolic factors are known to affect the function of small blood vessels (endothelial dysfunction), as well as lumen size. The larger lesions were more strongly associated with low-density lipoprotein cholesterol. The latter is a risk factor linked with large vessel atherosclerosis. Both types of lesions shared the common risk factors of advancing age, hypertension, and smoking. This distinction between the 2 forms of small vessel disease may explain why studies of lacunar infarcts differ with regard to whether diabetes is an underlying risk factor.

SUMMARY

In this brief review of atherosclerotic CVD in older diabetic adults, we have emphasized 4 points. First, although the relative risk for cardiovascular events and mortality seems to be less pronounced in older than in middle-aged adults, diabetes remains an important risk factor for these outcomes, particularly mortality, well into old age (ie, beyond age 70–74 years). Second, the presence of subclinical vascular disease is an important determinant of who develops and who does not develop clinical CVD. Third, newly detected diabetes poses a near-term risk of CVD. Finally, diabetes affects not only the large arteries of the brain, but the small arteries and arterioles as well.

REFERENCES

1. Psaty BM, Furberg CD, Kuller LH, et al. Traditional risk factors and subclinical disease measures as predictors of first myocardial infarction in older adults: the Cardiovascular Health Study. Arch Intern Med 1999;159:1339–47.
2. Kronmal RA, Barzilay JI, Smith NL, et al. Mortality in pharmacologically treated older adults with diabetes: the Cardiovascular Health Study, 1989–2001. PLoS Med 2006;3(10):e400.
3. Wingard DL, Barrett-Connor E. Heart disease and diabetes. In: Harris MI, Cowie CC, Stern MP, et al, editors. Diabetes in America. 2nd edition. Washington, DC: NIH Publication; 1995. p. 429–48, 95–1468. Available at: http://diabetes.niddk.nih.gov/dm/pubs/america/pdf/chapter19.pdf.
4. Geiss LS, Herman WH, Smith PJ. Mortality in non-insulin-dependent diabetes. In: Harris MI, Cowie CC, Stern MP, et al, editors. Diabetes in America. 2nd edition. Washington, DC: NIH Publication; 1995. p. 233–58, 95–1468. Available at: http://diabetes.niddk.nih.gov/dm/pubs/america/pdf/chapter11.pdf.
5. Bertoni AG, Krop JS, Anderson GF, et al. Diabetes-related morbidity and mortality in a national sample of U.S. elders. Diabetes Care 2002;25:471–5.
6. The Emerging Risk Factors Collaboration. Diabetes mellitus, fasting blood glucose concentration, and risk of vascular disease: a collaborative meta-analysis of 102 prospective studies. Lancet 2010;375:2215–22.
7. Barrett-Connor EL, Cohn BA, Wingard DL, et al. Why is diabetes mellitus a stronger risk factor for fatal ischemic heart disease in women than in men? The Rancho Bernardo Study. JAMA 1991;265:627–31.

8. Smith NL, Barzilay JI, Kronmal R, et al. New-onset diabetes and risk of all-cause and cardiovascular mortality: the Cardiovascular Health Study. Diabetes Care 2006;29:2012–7.
9. Haffner SM, Lehto S, Rönnemaa T, et al. Mortality from coronary heart disease in subjects with type 2 diabetes and in nondiabetic subjects with and without prior myocardial infarction. N Engl J Med 1998;339:229–34.
10. Carnethon MR, Biggs ML, Barzilay J, et al. Diabetes and coronary heart disease as risk factors for mortality in older adults. Am J Med 2010;123:556.e1–9.
11. Wannamethee SG, Shaper AG, Whincup PH, et al. Impact of diabetes on cardiovascular disease risk and all-cause mortality in older men. Arch Intern Med 2011; 171:404–10.
12. Giorda CB, Avogaro A, Maggini M, et al, Diabetes and Informatics Study Group. Recurrence of cardiovascular events in patients with type 2 diabetes: epidemiology and risk factors. Diabetes Care 2008;31:2154–9.
13. Strandberg TE, Pitkala KH, Berglind S, et al. Multifactorial intervention to prevent recurrent cardiovascular events in patients 75 years or older: the Drugs and Evidence-Based Medicine in the Elderly (DEBATE) study: a randomized, controlled trial. Am Heart J 2006;152:585–92.
14. Koller MT, Leening MJ, Wolbers M, et al. Development and validation of a coronary risk prediction model for older U.S. and European persons in the Cardiovascular Health Study and the Rotterdam Study. Ann Intern Med 2012;157:389–97.
15. Kuller LH, Velentgas P, Barzilay J, et al. Diabetes mellitus: subclinical cardiovascular disease and risk of incident cardiovascular disease and all-cause mortality. Arterioscler Thromb Vasc Biol 2000;20:823–9.
16. Kuller L, Borhani N, Furberg C, et al. Prevalence of subclinical atherosclerosis and cardiovascular disease and association with risk factors in the Cardiovascular Health Study. Am J Epidemiol 1994;139:1164–79.
17. Goldberg RB, Mellies MJ, Sacks FM, et al, for the CARE investigators. Cardiovascular events and their reduction with pravastatin in diabetic and glucose-intolerant myocardial infarction survivors with average cholesterol levels: subgroup analyses in the cholesterol and recurrent events. Circulation 1998;98: 2513–9.
18. Barzilay JI, Spiekerman CF, Kuller LH, et al. Prevalence of clinical and isolated subclinical cardiovascular disease in older adults with glucose disorders. The Cardiovascular Health Study. Diabetes Care 2001;24:1233–9.
19. Metter EJ, Windham BG, Maggio M, et al. Glucose and insulin measurements from the oral glucose tolerance test and mortality prediction. Diabetes Care 2008;31:1026–30.
20. Barzilay JI, Spiekerman CF, Wahl PW, et al. Cardiovascular disease in older adults with glucose disorders: comparison of American Diabetes Association criteria for diabetes mellitus with WHO criteria. Lancet 1999;354:622–5.
21. Smith NL, Barzilay JI, Shaffer D, et al. Fasting and 2-hour postchallenge serum glucose measures and risk of incident cardiovascular events in the elderly: the Cardiovascular Health Study. Arch Intern Med 2002;162:209–16.
22. Barrett-Connor E, Ferrara A. Isolated postchallenge hyperglycemia and the risk of fatal cardiovascular disease in older women and men. The Rancho Bernardo Study. Diabetes Care 1998;21:1236–9.
23. Glucose tolerance and mortality: comparison of WHO and American Diabetes Association diagnostic criteria. The DECODE study group. European Diabetes Epidemiology Group. Diabetes Epidemiology: Collaborative analysis of Diagnostic criteria in Europe. Lancet 1999;354(9179):617–21.

24. Kuller LH. Stroke and diabetes. In: Harris MI, Cowie CC, Stern MP, et al, editors. Diabetes in America. 2nd edition. Washington, DC: NIH Publication; 1995. p. 449–56, 95–1468. Available at: http://diabetes.niddk.nih.gov/dm/pubs/america/pdf/chapter20.pdf.

25. Gray CS, Scott JF, French JM, et al. Prevalence and prediction of unrecognised diabetes mellitus and impaired glucose tolerance following acute stroke. Age Ageing 2004;33:71–7.

26. Fox CS, Coady S, Sorlie PD, et al. Increasing cardiovascular disease burden due to diabetes mellitus: the Framingham Heart Study. Circulation 2007;115:1544–50.

27. Longstreth WT Jr, Bernick C, Manolio TA, et al. Lacunar infarcts defined by magnetic resonance imaging of 3660 elderly people: the Cardiovascular Health Study. Arch Neurol 1998;55:1217–25.

28. Longstreth WT Jr, Dulberg C, Manolio TA, et al. Incidence, manifestations, and predictors of brain infarcts defined by serial cranial magnetic resonance imaging in the elderly: the Cardiovascular Health Study. Stroke 2002;33:2376–82.

29. Vermeer SE, Deb Heijer T, Koudstaal PJ, et al, Rotterdam Scan Study. Incidence and risk factors of silent brain infarcts in the population-based Rotterdam Scan Study. Stroke 2003;34:392–6.

30. Bezerra DC, Sharrett AR, Matsushita K, et al. Risk factors for lacune subtypes in the Atherosclerosis Risk in Communities (ARIC) Study. Neurology 2012;78:102–8.

The Effect of Type 2 Diabetes on Body Composition of Older Adults

Annemarie Koster, PhD[a],*, Laura A. Schaap, PhD[b]

KEYWORDS

- Diabetes mellitus • Body composition • Body fat distribution • Muscle mass
- Older adults

KEY POINTS

- Type 2 diabetes is associated with more visceral fat, less thigh subcutaneous fat, and more fat infiltration in muscle compared with persons without diabetes.
- Older adults with type 2 diabetes show accelerated decline of muscle mass.
- People with undiagnosed/untreated type 2 diabetes are at particularly high risk of unfavorable changes in fat mass and lean mass.
- Future studies are needed to examine the consequences of the changes in body composition in patients with type 2 diabetes on physical functioning, morbidity, and risk of mortality.

INTRODUCTION

The prevalence of type 2 diabetes has increased dramatically over the past decades and will continue to increase worldwide.[1] This increase is due to demographic changes such as aging and shifts toward an unhealthy lifestyle, including physical inactivity and obesity. Body weight is a well-established risk factor for type 2 diabetes.[2] Not only total adiposity but also fat distribution is important; visceral fat in particular is strongly associated with insulin resistance and glucose intolerance, and increased visceral adiposity predicts incident diabetes.[3,4] By contrast, subcutaneous fat in the lower body, often measured by hip circumference, may be protective against metabolic diseases such as type 2 diabetes.[5–7] An unfavorable body composition not only can be a cause of type 2 diabetes but also may be the consequence of the

Disclosure Statement: The authors disclose no conflict of interest.
[a] Department of Social Medicine, CAPHRI School for Public Health and Primary Care, Maastricht University, PO Box 616, 6200 MD Maastricht, The Netherlands; [b] Department of Health Sciences, Faculty of Earth and Life Sciences, VU University Amsterdam, de Boelelaan 1085, 1081 HV, Amsterdam, The Netherlands
* Corresponding author.
E-mail address: a.koster@maastrichtuniversity.nl

Clin Geriatr Med 31 (2015) 41–49
http://dx.doi.org/10.1016/j.cger.2014.08.020
0749-0690/15/$ – see front matter © 2015 Elsevier Inc. All rights reserved.
geriatric.theclinics.com

disease. This review focuses on observational studies of type 2 diabetes and its consequences for fat mass, fat distribution, and lean mass in older adults, and changes in these parameters.

AGING AND CHANGES IN BODY COMPOSITION

Aging is associated with changes in body composition, in that fat mass generally increases with age while lean mass decreases.[8–11] The increases in total fat mass and the progressive loss of lean mass are independent of changes in weight.[11,12] Older people tend to gain fat mass into early old age, while fat mass decreases in late old age. The Health, Aging, and Body Composition (Health ABC) study showed that a large group of well-functioned men and women aged 70 to 79 years lost weight gradually, while still gaining fat mass until the age of 75.[13] After age 75, the participants started to lose weight more rapidly, accompanied by a loss of fat mass. A linear decline of lean mass was found.

In addition to the changes in total fat mass with age, there is also redistribution of fat mass over the different fat depots.[14] Subcutaneous adipose tissue seems to decrease with age, while visceral fat, liver fat, and intermuscular fat increase.[14] Fat storage in these depots has been strongly associated with metabolic disturbances. Together, the age-related changes in body composition are associated with increased risk of morbidity and disability.[15,16]

DIABETES AND FAT DISTRIBUTION

Although it is generally known that type 2 diabetes is associated with overweight and obesity,[17] knowledge about fat distribution and changes therein in persons with type 2 diabetes is limited. Several small case-control studies among middle-aged persons found either no differences in fat distribution[18–20] or an unfavorable fat distribution with more truncal fat and less peripheral fat in persons with type 2 diabetes compared with healthy controls.[21,22]

Fat distribution in older adults with type 2 diabetes was examined in a small case-control study.[23] This study found no differences in total body fat between women with type 2 diabetes (n = 42, mean age 64 years) and healthy age-matched and body mass index (BMI)-matched controls (n = 42), but did show that the women with diabetes had significantly less lower body fat (measured by dual-energy X-ray absorptiometry [DXA]) than the control group.[23] Using data from the Look AHEAD trial, which included both middle-aged and older adults, Azuma and colleagues[24] examined fat distribution in 67 obese persons (mean age 60) with type 2 diabetes and 35 healthy obese persons, using DXA and CT. The study showed that trunk fat mass was significantly larger in persons with type 2 diabetes than in healthy persons. Furthermore, persons with type 2 diabetes had less leg fat mass (-1.2 ± 0.4 kg), more subfascial adipose tissue (3.2 ± 1.6 cm^2), and a lower liver CT attenuation (-7 ± 3 HU), indicating a higher fat content within the liver. Muscle attenuation was also lower in persons with type 2 diabetes (-2 ± 1 HU), but this was no longer significant after adjustment for sex, age, race, study site, height, and fat mass. In another study from the Look AHEAD trial, Gallagher and colleagues[25] compared body composition between persons with type 2 diabetes (56 women and 37 men) and matched controls, using whole-body MRI. Unlike DXA, MRI can discriminate between adipose tissue subdepots. The study found that women with type 2 diabetes had less total adipose tissue, while men with type 2 diabetes had more total adipose tissue compared with controls. Considerable differences in fat distribution were, however, found between persons with type 2 diabetes and controls in both men and women. Visceral adipose tissue mass was greater in persons with type 2 diabetes, especially in white persons compared with African Americans; the reason for this race difference was unknown. Furthermore, persons with type 2 diabetes had more intermuscular adipose tissue than controls, and this difference became larger at higher levels of adiposity. In contrast, persons with type 2 diabetes had less thigh subcutaneous adipose tissue than the control group, and this difference was greater in white persons. In view of the small sample size of this study (especially the subgroups based on sex and race), more studies are needed to confirm these findings.

A few larger observational studies have examined fat distribution in older persons with type 2 diabetes. Data from the Health ABC Study revealed that intermuscular fat mass (measured by CT) was larger in persons with type 2 diabetes (11.2 ± 9.4 cm^2 for men, 12.1± 6.1 cm^2 in women) compared with persons with normal glucose tolerance (9.2 ± 5.9 cm^2 for men, 9.4 ± 5.3 cm^2 for women), after adjustment for the proportion of total body fat.[26] Visceral fat was also higher in men and women with type 2 diabetes (172 ± 79 vs 145 ± 66 cm^2 for men, 162 ± 66 vs 116 ± 54 cm^2 for women).[26] Another study from Health ABC used a nested case-control design to examine the association between fat and type 2 diabetes and found that increased levels of visceral fat were associated with a 3-fold increased risk of diabetes in women and a 30% increased risk of diabetes in men, after adjustment for BMI.[27] Heshka and colleagues[28] investigated body composition differences between persons with type 2 diabetes (n = 1318) and healthy controls (n = 242) using DXA in a large sample from the Look AHEAD trial. After adjustment for weight, height, age, sex, and race, total fat mass was smaller (∼1.4 kg) in persons with type 2 diabetes than in healthy persons. Persons with type 2 diabetes had more fat in the arms and trunk compared with healthy persons, but had less fat in the legs.

Longitudinal studies that focused on changes in fat mass and fat distribution in type 2 diabetes have been scarce. Park and colleagues[29] examined annual changes in body composition in persons with type 2 diabetes (undiagnosed and diagnosed) and persons without diabetes, aged 70 and older. This study found an annual loss of total body mass in all 3 groups (−193 ± 22 g/y in persons without diabetes, −435 ± 79 g/y in persons with undiagnosed diabetes, and −293 ± 72 g/y in persons with diagnosed diabetes). Persons with diabetes gradually lost trunk fat (−39 ± 35 g/y in undiagnosed diabetes, −34 ± 32 g/y in diagnosed diabetes), as well as appendicular fat (−51 ± 24 g/y in persons with undiagnosed diabetes, −27 ± 24 g/y in persons with diagnosed diabetes). There was also a loss of total fat mass in persons with type 2 diabetes (−94 ± 53 g/y in those with undiagnosed diabetes, −66 ± 53 g/y in diagnosed diabetes), while persons without diabetes showed an increase in fat mass of 25 g/y. After adjustment for the change in body weight, there was a significant relative annual increase in trunk fat (96 ± 14 g/y) in persons with diagnosed diabetes and a significant relative annual increase in appendicular fat (73 ± 14 g/y) in persons with undiagnosed diabetes, while persons without diabetes showed a greater increase in trunk fat (125 ± 5 g/y) and a smaller increase in appendicular fat (41 ± 4 g/y). Total fat mass increased in all 3 groups, without significant differences across the groups (160 ± 20 g/y, 203 ± 23 g/y, 163 ± 7 g/y in persons with diabetes, persons with undiagnosed diabetes, and persons without diabetes, respectively). These data show that although all 3 groups lost body mass, body composition changed unfavorably, with a relative increase in total body fat and trunk fat mass.

In a large study of more than 3000 Chinese adults aged 65 and older, diabetes was associated with a significantly greater loss of body mass over a period of 4 years in age-adjusted analyses (2.3% loss in men with diabetes compared with 0.9% loss in men without diabetes and 2.4% loss in women with diabetes compared with 1.2% loss in women without diabetes).[30] Men with diabetes also showed a greater total body fat loss than men without diabetes. In the Osteoporotic Fractures in Men (MrOS) study, the association between insulin resistance and changes in body composition over a period of 4.6 years in more than 3000 older men without type 2 diabetes was examined.[31] This study reported that men who were the most insulin-resistant had higher baseline body weight and fat mass. The most insulin-resistant men were more likely to lose weight of 5% or more (odds ratio [OR] 1.88; 1.46–2.43) and were less likely to gain 5% or more total (OR 0.56; 0.45–0.68) or truncal fat mass (OR 0.52; 0.42–0.64).[31] In the same study population, men with untreated diabetes or diabetes treated without insulin sensitizers had the greatest loss in weight and total fat mass compared with normoglycemic men in unadjusted analyses (−2.8% vs −1.2% change in weight and −1.9% vs +1.2% change in fat mass).[32] In 2 of the above-mentioned longitudinal studies, only crude effects on fat mass were reported[30,32]; this makes it difficult to draw conclusions about the association between type 2 diabetes and change in fat mass.

DIABETES AND MUSCLE MASS

Cross-sectional studies indicate that older adults with type 2 diabetes have a higher muscle mass because of a higher body weight. In the Health ABC Study, participants with type 2 diabetes had more lean mass, as assessed by DXA, in the arms and legs than participants without the disease, which was due to differences in body weight.[33] Muscle quality, defined as muscle strength divided by muscle mass, was significantly lower in participants with type 2 diabetes.[33] A study among a small sample of the Look AHEAD trial found no significant difference in fat-free mass, assessed by DXA, or muscle area, assessed by CT, between 67 persons with and 35 without type 2 diabetes.[24] Data from more than 1500 participants of the Look AHEAD trial indicated that compared with controls, participants with type 2 diabetes had 0.6 kg more lean mass in the trunk and 0.5 kg less lean mass in the leg.[28] A recent study among 60 older adults showed that, compared with age-matched normoglycemic controls, older adults with type 2 diabetes had an approximately 3% lower leg lean mass and appendicular lean mass; body weight was similar in both groups.[34] The study also involved taking muscle biopsy samples and found no differences in fiber-size or fiber-type distribution between the 2 groups. The Korean Sarcopenic Obesity Study, which included 810 subjects (414 persons with type 2 diabetes and 396 controls), examined the prevalence of sarcopenia.[35] The prevalence of sarcopenia, defined as a skeletal muscle index less than 2 SDs below the mean value of a young reference group, was significantly higher in men and women aged 60 and older with diabetes than in those without diabetes (19.0% vs 5.1% in men and 27.0% vs 14.0% in women).[35] In the Korea National Health and Nutrition Examination Survey, with nonobese participants aged 60 and older, sarcopenic subjects had a higher prevalence of diabetes than participants without sarcopenia (32.9% vs 17.3%).[36]

Longitudinal studies have found that older adults with type 2 diabetes show a more rapid decline of lean mass than normoglycemic participants. Using data from the Health ABC study, Park and colleagues[37] were the first to show in a large observational cohort study that men and women with type 2 diabetes lost greater amounts of leg lean mass than those without diabetes over a period of 3 years of follow-up (−0.29 ± 0.03 kg vs −0.23 ± 0.01 kg). In a follow-up article from the Health ABC Study, those with type 2 diabetes showed an excessive loss of appendicular lean mass (−130 ± 11 g/y vs −113 ± 4 g/y), as measured by DXA over a period of 5 years of follow-up, compared with participants without type 2 diabetes.[29] The loss of muscle mass was especially apparent in previously undiagnosed cases (−149 g/y appendicular lean mass), which were participants newly diagnosed with type 2 diabetes based on an oral glucose tolerance test. This finding suggests that the most rapid decline in muscle mass takes place in the early stages of the disease or when diabetes is untreated in older adults. This study also assessed the change in thigh muscle mass assessed by CT and showed that women with type 2 diabetes showed about a 2-fold greater loss of thigh muscle mass than their nondiabetic counterparts (−10.0 ± 1.1 cm² vs −5.3 ± 0.4 cm²) adjusted for baseline body weight and changes in body weight. No significant differences in the loss of thigh muscle were found between diabetic and nondiabetic men.[29]

A study among 3153 Chinese adults aged 65 years and older showed that participants with diabetes lost a significantly greater amount of lean mass and in particular appendicular lean mass over a period of 4 years than those without diabetes (−3.0% vs −1.5% in men and −3.4% vs 1.9% in women).[30] This association was independent of age, smoking, physical activity, and diabetes-related conditions, including low ankle-brachial index, high BMI, heart disease, stroke, and hypertension. Similar to the findings of the Health ABC study, the absolute amount of lean mass was greater in men and women with diabetes,[38] whereas the ratio of appendicular lean mass to total lean mass was lower in participants with diabetes.[30]

The MrOS study examined the association between insulin resistance and changes in body composition in men without type 2 diabetes (n = 3132). This study reported that men with the greatest insulin resistance had higher baseline lean mass but lost more total and appendicular lean mass over a period of 4.6 years of follow-up than the most insulin-sensitive men.[31] The most insulin-resistant men (highest quartile of HOMA-IR) had a significantly increased odds of losing 5% or more total lean mass (OR 2.09; 1.60–2.73) and appendicular lean mass (OR 1.57; 1.27–1.95) than men in the lowest quartile of HOMA-IR. In the same study, a greater loss of total and appendicular lean mass was observed in men with untreated diabetes than in normoglycemic men (−2.5% vs −1.9% change in total lean mass and −4.2% vs −3.0% change in appendicular lean mass).[32] In addition, those with diabetes treated without insulin sensitizers lost more lean mass than normoglycemic men (−2.9% vs −1.9 change in total lean mass and −4.4% vs −3.0% change in appendicular lean mass). Men with diabetes who were treated with insulin sensitizers lost significantly less lean mass than their normoglycemic counterparts (−1.1% vs −1.9 change in total lean mass and −1.8% vs −3.0% change in appendicular lean mass).[32] In a study among 142 renal replacement therapy patients, those with type 2 diabetes show an accelerated loss of lean body mass as compared with patients without diabetes over a period of 1 year.[39]

SUMMARY

The results of the observational studies on fat distribution discussed allow the conclusion that type 2 diabetes is associated with an unfavorable body composition, characterized by more visceral fat, less thigh subcutaneous fat, and more fat infiltration in the muscle than persons without type 2 diabetes. Few longitudinal studies have examined the effect of type 2 diabetes on changes in fat mass, and type 2 diabetes in old age seems associated with greater loss of fat mass. Although cross-sectional studies do not show a clear association between type 2 diabetes and muscle mass, longitudinal studies clearly show an accelerated decline in muscle mass in older adults with type 2 diabetes compared with those without diabetes.

Little is known about the impact of these longitudinal changes in body composition in older adults with diabetes on subsequent health outcomes, including functional limitations and disability, which should be subject for future studies. A recent systematic review and meta-analysis shows that obesity, a large waist circumference, and a high percentage of body fat were associated with increased risk of functional decline. In addition, poor muscle strength was associated with functional decline, whereas low muscle mass was not significant.[15,16] A recent study investigating the independent associations between changes in body composition and gait speed shows that increasing intermuscular fat and decreasing thigh muscle were important predictors of gait speed decline.[40] Although there are very few studies, age-related loss of muscle mass may also increase risk of mortality.[16]

The loss of fat mass and lean mass is especially marked in older adults with undiagnosed or untreated type 2 diabetes,[29,32] which underlines the need for early detection of the disease. Diabetes treatment is important and diabetes medication also affects body composition.[32,41–43] For most types of medication, the effect on weight (either weight gain or weight stability) is evident.[43,44] The effects on specific body composition measures such as muscle mass are largely unknown, although one study found that patients treated with insulin sensitizers (metformin and/or thiazolidinediones) show less decline in muscle mass than untreated patients.[32] Another explanation for the particularly unfavorable changes in body composition in those with undiagnosed diabetes compared with those with diagnosed type 2 diabetes could be the lifestyle recommendations that persons receive from their physician after diagnosis. Patients with diabetes are usually recommended to increase their physical activity levels and to change their diet.[45] Adherence to these lifestyle recommendations will likely have a positive effect on their body composition. Pharmacologic treatment of type 2 diabetes together with lifestyle changes may be important in preventing unfavorable changes in body composition and the associated health consequences.

Several mechanisms have been suggested to be responsible for the association between type 2 diabetes and accelerated loss of muscle mass. Type 2 diabetes is characterized by insulin resistance and impaired insulin secretion by the pancreas. Insulin resistance causes a reduced insulin-mediated glucose uptake in skeletal muscle,[46] resulting in reduced energy production and weaker contraction of the muscle, especially of type I fibers,[47] which are more common in the muscle of older persons than type II fibers.[48] Furthermore, insulin resistance may lead to muscle protein breakdown.[49] Another possible mechanism may be the increase in inflammatory markers that occurs during aging. Studies have suggested that chronic inflammation is associated with insulin resistance,[50,51] which could in turn result in impaired insulin action on muscle protein metabolism. Fat mass loss in type 2 diabetes might be explained by impaired insulin action, which accelerates adipose tissue lipolysis.[52]

In conclusion, type 2 diabetes in old age is associated with unfavorable changes in body composition, in particular, the accelerated loss of lean mass. More prospective studies are needed to understand the impact of type 2 diabetes on changes in fat mass and fat distribution, because current evidence is limited. In studies examining the association between diabetes and changes in body composition, it is very important to distinguish between persons with diagnosed diabetes and those with undiagnosed/untreated diabetes, as the latter seem to be at particularly high risk of unfavorable changes in fat mass and lean mass. Finally, future studies are needed to understand the health consequences of changes in body composition with type 2 diabetes.

REFERENCES

1. Whiting DR, Guariguata L, Weil C, et al. IDF diabetes atlas: global estimates of the prevalence of diabetes for 2011 and 2030. Diabetes Res Clin Pract 2011; 94(3):311–21.
2. Mokdad AH, Ford ES, Bowman BA, et al. Prevalence of obesity, diabetes, and obesity-related health risk factors, 2001. JAMA 2003;289(1):76–9.
3. Boyko EJ, Fujimoto WY, Leonetti DL, et al. Visceral adiposity and risk of type 2 diabetes: a prospective study among Japanese Americans. Diabetes Care 2000;23(4):465–71.
4. Neeland IJ, Turer AT, Ayers CR, et al. Dysfunctional adiposity and the risk of prediabetes and type 2 diabetes in obese adults. JAMA 2012;308(11):1150–9.
5. Janghorbani M, Momeni F, Dehghani M. Hip circumference, height and risk of type 2 diabetes: systematic review and meta-analysis. Obes Rev 2012;13(12): 1172–81.
6. Snijder MB, Visser M, Dekker JM, et al. Low subcutaneous thigh fat is a risk factor for unfavourable glucose and lipid levels, independently of high abdominal fat. The Health ABC Study. Diabetologia 2005;48(2):301–8.
7. Snijder MB, Dekker JM, Visser M, et al. Associations of hip and thigh circumferences independent of waist circumference with the incidence of type 2 diabetes: the Hoorn Study. Am J Clin Nutr 2003;77(5):1192–7.
8. Delmonico MJ, Harris TB, Visser M, et al. Longitudinal study of muscle strength, quality, and adipose tissue infiltration. Am J Clin Nutr 2009;90(6):1579–85.
9. Hughes VA, Frontera WR, Roubenoff R, et al. Longitudinal changes in body composition in older men and women: role of body weight change and physical activity. Am J Clin Nutr 2002;76(2):473–81.
10. Newman AB, Lee JS, Visser M, et al. Weight change and the conservation of lean mass in old age: the Health, Aging and Body Composition Study. Am J Clin Nutr 2005;82(4):872–8.
11. Gallagher D, Ruts E, Visser M, et al. Weight stability masks sarcopenia in elderly men and women. Am J Physiol Endocrinol Metab 2000;279(2):E366–75.
12. Zamboni M, Zoico E, Scartezzini T, et al. Body composition changes in stable-weight elderly subjects: the effect of sex. Aging Clin Exp Res 2003;15(4):321–7.
13. Koster A, Visser M, Simonsick EM, et al. Association between fitness and changes in body composition and muscle strength. J Am Geriatr Soc 2010; 58(2):219–26.
14. Kuk JL, Saunders TJ, Davidson LE, et al. Age-related changes in total and regional fat distribution. Ageing Res Rev 2009;8(4):339–48.
15. Schaap LA, Koster A, Visser M. Adiposity, muscle mass, and muscle strength in relation to functional decline in older persons. Epidemiol Rev 2013;35(1):51–65.
16. Visser M, Schaap LA. Consequences of sarcopenia. Clin Geriatr Med 2011; 27(3):387–99.
17. Qiao Q, Nyamdorj R. Is the association of type II diabetes with waist circumference or waist-to-hip ratio stronger than that with body mass index? Eur J Clin Nutr 2010;64(1):30–4.
18. Svendsen OL, Hassager C. Body composition and fat distribution measured by dual-energy x-ray absorptiometry in premenopausal and postmenopausal insulin-dependent and non-insulin-dependent diabetes mellitus patients. Metabolism 1998;47(2):212–6.
19. Maiolo C, Mohamed EI, Di DN, et al. Body composition and pulmonary function in obese type 2 diabetic women. Diabetes Nutr Metab 2002;15(1):20–5.

20. Poynten AM, Markovic TP, Maclean EL, et al. Fat oxidation, body composition and insulin sensitivity in diabetic and normoglycaemic obese adults 5 years after weight loss. Int J Obes Relat Metab Disord 2003;27(10):1212–8.

21. Abate N, Garg A, Peshock RM, et al. Relationship of generalized and regional adiposity to insulin sensitivity in men with NIDDM. Diabetes 1996;45(12): 1684–93.

22. Bavenholm PN, Kuhl J, Pigon J, et al. Insulin resistance in type 2 diabetes: association with truncal obesity, impaired fitness, and atypical malonyl coenzyme A regulation. J Clin Endocrinol Metab 2003;88(1):82–7.

23. Stoney RM, Walker KZ, Best JD, et al. Do postmenopausal women with NIDDM have a reduced capacity to deposit and conserve lower-body fat? Diabetes Care 1998;21(5):828–30.

24. Azuma K, Heilbronn LK, Albu JB, et al. Adipose tissue distribution in relation to insulin resistance in type 2 diabetes mellitus. Am J Physiol Endocrinol Metab 2007;293(1):E435–42.

25. Gallagher D, Kelley DE, Yim JE, et al. Adipose tissue distribution is different in type 2 diabetes. Am J Clin Nutr 2009;89(3):807–14.

26. Goodpaster BH, Krishnaswami S, Resnick H, et al. Association between regional adipose tissue distribution and both type 2 diabetes and impaired glucose tolerance in elderly men and women. Diabetes Care 2003;26(2):372–9.

27. Kanaya AM, Harris T, Goodpaster BH, et al. Adipocytokines attenuate the association between visceral adiposity and diabetes in older adults. Diabetes Care 2004;27(6):1375–80.

28. Heshka S, Ruggiero A, Bray GA, et al. Altered body composition in type 2 diabetes mellitus. Int J Obes (Lond) 2008;32(5):780–7.

29. Park SW, Goodpaster BH, Lee JS, et al. Excessive loss of skeletal muscle mass in older adults with type 2 diabetes. Diabetes Care 2009;32(11):1993–7.

30. Lee JS, Auyeung TW, Leung J, et al. The effect of diabetes mellitus on age-associated lean mass loss in 3153 older adults. Diabet Med 2010;27(12): 1366–71.

31. Lee CG, Boyko EJ, Strotmeyer ES, et al. Association between insulin resistance and lean mass loss and fat mass gain in older men without diabetes mellitus. J Am Geriatr Soc 2011;59(7):1217–24.

32. Lee CG, Boyko EJ, Barrett-Connor E, et al. Insulin sensitizers may attenuate lean mass loss in older men with diabetes. Diabetes Care 2011;34(11):2381–6.

33. Park SW, Goodpaster BH, Strotmeyer ES, et al. Decreased muscle strength and quality in older adults with type 2 diabetes: the health, aging, and body composition study. Diabetes 2006;55(6):1813–8.

34. Leenders M, Verdijk LB, van der Hoeven L, et al. Patients with type 2 diabetes show a greater decline in muscle mass, muscle strength, and functional capacity with aging. J Am Med Dir Assoc 2013;14(8):585–92.

35. Kim TN, Park MS, Yang SJ, et al. Prevalence and determinant factors of sarcopenia in patients with type 2 diabetes: the Korean Sarcopenic Obesity Study (KSOS). Diabetes Care 2010;33(7):1497–9.

36. Moon SS. Low skeletal muscle mass is associated with insulin resistance, diabetes, and metabolic syndrome in the Korean population: the Korea National Health and Nutrition Examination Survey (KNHANES) 2009-2010. Endocr J 2014;61(1):61–70.

37. Park SW, Goodpaster BH, Strotmeyer ES, et al. Accelerated loss of skeletal muscle strength in older adults with type 2 diabetes: the health, aging, and body composition study. Diabetes Care 2007;30(6):1507–12.

38. Lee JS, Auyeung TW, Kwok T, et al. Associated factors and health impact of sarcopenia in older Chinese men and women: a cross-sectional study. Gerontology 2007;53(6):404–10.
39. Pupim LB, Heimburger O, Qureshi AR, et al. Accelerated lean body mass loss in incident chronic dialysis patients with diabetes mellitus. Kidney Int 2005;68(5):2368–74.
40. Beavers KM, Beavers DP, Houston DK, et al. Associations between body composition and gait-speed decline: results from the Health, Aging, and Body Composition study. Am J Clin Nutr 2013;97(3):552–60.
41. Virtanen KA, Hallsten K, Parkkola R, et al. Differential effects of rosiglitazone and metformin on adipose tissue distribution and glucose uptake in type 2 diabetic subjects. Diabetes 2003;52(2):283–90.
42. Stumvoll M, Nurjhan N, Perriello G, et al. Metabolic effects of metformin in non-insulin-dependent diabetes mellitus. N Engl J Med 1995;333(9):550–4.
43. Meneghini LF, Orozco-Beltran D, Khunti K, et al. Weight beneficial treatments for type 2 diabetes. J Clin Endocrinol Metab 2011;96(11):3337–53.
44. Pedersen SD. Impact of newer medications for type 2 diabetes on body weight. Curr Obes Rep 2013;2(2):134–41.
45. American Diabetes Association. Standards of medical care in diabetes–2014. Diabetes Care 2014;37(Suppl 1):S14–80.
46. Pendergrass M, Bertoldo A, Bonadonna R, et al. Muscle glucose transport and phosphorylation in type 2 diabetic, obese nondiabetic, and genetically predisposed individuals. Am J Physiol Endocrinol Metab 2007;292(1):E92–100.
47. Abbatecola AM, Paolisso G, Fattoretti P, et al. Discovering pathways of sarcopenia in older adults: a role for insulin resistance on mitochondria dysfunction. J Nutr Health Aging 2011;15(10):890–5.
48. Song XM, Ryder JW, Kawano Y, et al. Muscle fiber type specificity in insulin signal transduction. Am J Physiol 1999;277(6 Pt 2):R1690–6.
49. Pereira S, Marliss EB, Morais JA, et al. Insulin resistance of protein metabolism in type 2 diabetes. Diabetes 2008;57(1):56–63.
50. Marette A. Mediators of cytokine-induced insulin resistance in obesity and other inflammatory settings. Curr Opin Clin Nutr Metab Care 2002;5(4):377–83.
51. Wellen KE, Hotamisligil GS. Inflammation, stress, and diabetes. J Clin Invest 2005;115(5):1111–9.
52. Magkos F, Wang X, Mittendorfer B. Metabolic actions of insulin in men and women. Nutrition 2010;26(7–8):686–93.

Physical Function and Disability in Older Adults with Diabetes

Nathalie de Rekeneire, MD, MS[a],*, Stefano Volpato, MD, MPH[b]

KEYWORDS

- Diabetes • Functional limitation • Disability • Muscle strength • Aging

KEY POINTS

- Diabetes is associated with an excessive risk of developing functional limitation and disability.
- Disability can be defined in different ways, including difficulties with activities of daily living or with instrumental activities of daily living, and mobility limitations, whereas functional limitations are predominantly assessed by objectively measured physical performance.
- Diabetes increases the risk of disabling disorders such as cardiovascular disease, peripheral vascular disease, neuropathy, retinopathy, renal failure, cognitive decline, and depression. These disabling conditions do not totally explain the excess risk of disability associated with diabetes.
- The role of glycemic control and diabetes duration in this excess disability risk has shown conflicting results.
- Declines in muscle strength and muscle quality are potential mediators of the association between diabetes with functional decline and disability.

INTRODUCTION

Physical function is critical to maintaining independence and social interaction in the later years of life and is an important public health issue.[1] Functional decline and physical disability are common in older persons. According to the National Health and Nutrition Examination Surveys (NHANES), among people aged 80 and older 50% reported disability in instrumental activities of daily living (IADL), 27% in basic activities

Disclosure Statement: The authors disclose no conflict of interest.
[a] Section of Geriatrics, Department of Internal Medicine, Yale School of Medicine, 367 Cedar Street, Harkness Building A, Room 317A, New Haven, CT 06520, USA; [b] Section of Internal Medicine, Gerontology and Clinical, Nutrition, Department of Medical Sciences, Azienda Ospedaliero-Universitaria di Ferrara U.O. Medicina Interna Universitaria, University of Ferrara, Via Aldo Moro 8, 1B1 Stanza 1.35.30, Ferrara 44124, Italy
* Corresponding author.
E-mail address: nathalie.derekeneire@yale.edu

Clin Geriatr Med 31 (2015) 51–65
http://dx.doi.org/10.1016/j.cger.2014.08.018
0749-0690/15/$ – see front matter © 2015 Elsevier Inc. All rights reserved.

of daily living (ADL), and more than 35% in mobility activities.[2] The major underlying causes of physical disability are chronic diseases, both acute events, such as hip fracture and stroke, and slowly progressive diseases, including, but not limited to, arthritis, congestive heart failure, and diabetes. Furthermore, comorbidity, particularly certain combinations of chronic diseases, is also a strong risk factor for disability in itself.[3]

Diabetes prevalence increases as the population ages, with older aduts accounting for 30% of the adult population with diabetes in Western countries.[4] The multisystemic detrimental effect of diabetes interacts with several age-related pathophysiological changes generating disparate clinical pictures and complications.[5] In the last 20 years different epidemiologic and clinical investigations conducted in the geriatric population have consistently related diabetes with increased prevalence and incidence of disability in different domains of physical function.[6]

Understanding the relationship between diabetes and disability and elucidating the underlying biological mechanisms is important for patients and health care systems. For older patients with diabetes, disability and loss of independence may be of more concern than the traditional chronic complications. Therefore, prevention of disability could be a primary goal for patients, caregivers, physicians, and health organizations. This article describes the most compelling evidence for the association between diabetes and functional decline and disability and analyzes the potential explanatory biological mechanisms, focusing particularly on decline in muscle strength and quality.

FUNCTIONAL LIMITATION AND DISABILITY

The disablement model conceptualized by Nagi[7] defined functional limitation as "limitation in performance at the level of the whole organism or person"; whereas disability represents the presence of "limitation in performance of socially defined roles and tasks within a sociocultural and physical environment." The pathway to disability begins with a pathologic condition and impairments and then functional limitations are the intermediate steps leading to disability.

Functional limitations are strong predictors of disability, hospitalizations, nursing home admissions, and mortality.[8,9] Functional limitations are commonly evaluated with tests of physical performance using objective, standardized procedures. Gait speed evaluated over 4 m is among the most common physical performance test used in older adults. A usual gait speed less than 0.6 m/s is a predictor of risk for hospitalization and functional decline.[10] Another validated test widely used is the Short Physical Performance Battery (SPPB) that assesses lower-extremity physical performance.[11] The SPPB consists of timed tests of standing balance, a 4-m usual walk, and 5-chair stands; each test scoring 0 to 4 points. The SPPB score ranges from 0 to 12; a score of 12 showing higher performance.

Assessment of disability has included many different aspects of daily living activities representing self-care, instrumental, and mobility tasks. Disability can be defined as having a little, some, or much difficulty in doing such activities, or by the need for help for doing these activities.

ADL disability focuses on being able to perform basic self-care tasks such as bathing, dressing, transferring from bed to chair, toileting, grooming, and feeding oneself.

IADL disability refers to higher level daily living tasks. The IADL instrument explores the ability to use the telephone, shopping, food preparation, housekeeping, laundry, traveling, managing own medications, and managing finances.[12] Both ADL and IADL disability have been found to be significant predictors of nursing home admission[13,14] and mortality.[15]

Measuring the ability to walk a quarter mile (corresponding to 2–3 city blocks, or about 400 m) is an important element to consider for people living in the community. Inability or difficulty walking a quarter mile is a strong independent predictor of future ADL disability, health care utilization, and mortality.[16] Another common self-reported measure of mobility disability is the difficulty in climbing a flight of stairs.

DIABETES AND FUNCTIONAL LIMITATION

Most of the studies assessing the relationship between diabetes and functional limitation have been cross-sectional. Among 3300 nondisabled individuals examined at the sixth annual follow-up of the Established Populations for Epidemiologic Studies in the Elderly (EPESE) study, self-reported diabetes was associated with a 60% increase in the likelihood of a poorer SPPB score, independent of age, gender, and other comorbidities.[17] Data from a well-functioning population showed that, compared with those without diabetes, those with diabetes exhibited lower performance on objective measures of lower-extremity function that included walking speed, balance, and 5 chair stands.[18] Similar results on slower gait speed among older adults with diabetes in comparison to nondiabetic persons have been found in other studies, with altered and less efficient gait patterns in those with diabetes.[19–21]

Fewer studies have explored the longitudinal association between diabetes and physical performance. In the EPESE study, diabetes at baseline predicted increased risk of decline in physical performance by 10% to 60% over the 4 years of follow-up, independently of demographics and prevalent chronic conditions.[1] In the 3-year follow-up of the Women's Health and Aging Study (WHAS), a study of older women with baseline functional impairment or mild disability, women with diabetes exhibited greater additional decline in the SPPB than women without diabetes.[22] These findings have implications as poorer lower extremity performance, particularly gait speed, is more predictive of progressive and catastrophic ADL disability and mobility disability.[23]

DIABETES AND DISABILITY

Several cross-sectional and longitudinal studies among diverse populations have shown that diabetes is associated with disability, both for ADL and IADL disability and for mobility disability. Results from major epidemiologic studies are shown in **Table 1**.[1,22,24–31]

From a recent meta-analysis of cross-sectional data, diabetes was associated with higher risk of ADL disability (total pooled odds ratio [OR] of 1.87, 95% CI 1.66–2.10) and IADL disability (OR 1.67 [1.57–1.77]).[6] For example, in WHAS, women with diabetes had higher disability risk in ADL of 40%, and of 110% in IADL compared with women without diabetes.[24] In NHANES, comparable results were found; however, adjustment on demographic characteristics, hemoglobin A1c (HbA1c), diabetes duration, and comorbidities decreased the association to nonsignificance with an OR of 1.33 (0.84–2.09) and 1.08 (0.76–1.54) for ADL and IADL disability, respectively.[25]

Few longitudinal studies have explored this excessive disability risk associated with diabetes. In the EPESE study, of more than 6000 participants examined at the sixth annual follow-up, those with prevalent diabetes have twice the probability of having ADL disability.[1] Women with diabetes and mild to moderate disability at baseline have 60% risk of incident ADL disability over 3 years of follow-up.[22] The meta-analysis cited previously showed that, compared with those with no diabetes, people with diabetes were more likely to present incident ADL disability (pooled relative risk [RR] 1.82 [1.40–2.36]) and IADL disability (pooled RR 1.45 [1.20–1.75]).

Table 1
Major epidemiologic studies examining the risk of disability according to diabetes status instrumental activities of daily living or basic activities of daily living disability

	Study	Sex	Age	n	ADL (95% CI)	IADL (95% CI)	Adjustment Variables
ADL/IADL disability							
Cross-sectional studies							
Bourdel-Marchasson et al,[28] 1997	Paquid (1997)	Men/Women	≥65	2792	1.4 (0.9–1.9)	—	Unadjusted
Maty et al,[24] 2004	WHAS (2004)	Women	≥65	3570	1.4 (1.0–2.2)	2.1 (1.4–3.0)	Unadjusted
Maggi et al,[29] 2004	ILSA (2004)	Men	≥65	1912	1.2 (0.8–1.7)	—	Unadjusted
		Women		2586	1.7 (1.2–2.2)	—	
Kalyani et al,[25] 2010	NHANES (1999–2006)	Men/Women	≥60	6097	2.5 (2.0–3.2)	2.1 (1.7–2.7)	Demographic characteristics
Chau et al,[30] 2011	Elderly Health Centres	Men/Women	≥51	66,813	1.65 (1.51–1.80)	—	Demographic characteristics and education
Longitudinal studies							
Guralnik et al,[1] 1993	EPESE	Men	70–103	3046	2.0 (1.4–2.7)	—	Demographic characteristics, BMI, education, comorbidities
		Women		3935	1.7 (1.4–2.2)	—	
Volpato et al,[22] 2003	WHAS	Women	≥65	729	1.6 (1.2–2.1)	—	Demographic characteristics
Mobility disability							
Cross-sectional studies							
Guccione et al,[31] 1994	Framingham	Men/Women	≥60	1758	1.7 (1.1–2.7)	2.9 (1.5–5.8)	Demographic characteristics, comorbidities

Study		Men/Women	Age	N			
Bourdel-Marchasson et al,[28] 1997	Paquid	Men/Women	≥65	2792	1.8 (1.3–2.5)	1.7 (1.3–2.3)	Unadjusted
Gregg et al,[26] 2000	NHANES	Men Women	≥60	3113 3475	1.9 (1.3–2.6) 2.1 (1.5–2.9)	1.6 (1.1–2.4) 1.7 (1.5–2.9)	Demographic characteristics, education, BMI
Matty et al,[24] 2004	WHAS	Women	≥65	3570	+ Getting in or out of bed or chairs, and heavy housework 1.8 (1.3–2.5)		Demographic characteristics, education, comorbidities
Maggi et al,[29] 2004	ILSA	Men/Women	≥65	1912 2586	— —	1.9 (1.2–3.2) 1.5 (1.02–2.2)	Unadjusted
Longitudinal studies							
Guralnik et al,[1] 1993	EPESE	Men Women	70–103	3046 3935	1.6 (1.2–2.1) 1.7 (1.4–2.1)	1.4 (0.9–1.9) 1.7 (1.4–2.2)	Demographic characteristics, BMI, education, comorbidities
Gregg et al,[27] 2002	SOF	Women	≥65	8344	1.8 (1.4–2.2)	1.8 (1.4–2.3)	Demographic characteristics, education, BMI, physical activity, comorbidities
Volpato et al,[22] 2003	WHAS	Women	≥65	729	1.8 (1.3–2.5)	1.7 (1.3–2.3)	Age, race, smoking

Abbreviations: BMI, body mass index; ILSA, Italian Longitudinal Study of Aging; SOF, Study of Osteoporotic Fractures.

Pooled ORs from different cross-sectional studies showed that having diabetes was associated with an increased odds of mobility disability of 1.68 (1.50–1.88) compared with no diabetes.[6] In NHANES, both men and women with diabetes diagnosis reported difficulty in walking a quarter mile and climbing steps.[26] Women with diabetes had substantially higher odds of reporting much difficulty in walking (OR 1.94 [1.23–3.06]) and climbing steps (OR 1.83 [1.13–2.98]) than women without diabetes after full adjustment for demographic characteristics, education, and body mass index (BMI).

For longitudinal studies, results from the meta-analysis showed that people with diabetes were more likely to report incident mobility disability than those without diabetes (pooled RR 1·51, 95% CI 1.38–1.64). In the Study of Osteoporotic Fractures, women with diabetes had 76% higher risk of being unable to walk a quarter mile or climbing 10 steps after full adjustment for demographic characteristics, education, BMI, physical activity, and comorbidities.[27] Diabetes was also associated with an increased risk of 80% of incident mobility disability (walking quarter mile or climbing stairs) in women with diabetes compared with women with no diabetes.[22]

FACTORS EXPLAINING THE ASSOCIATION OF DIABETES WITH FUNCTIONAL LIMITATION AND DISABILITY

The association between diabetes and disability is quite complex because many impairments or comorbidities, related or not to diabetes, could intervene in the disablement process. **Figs. 1** and **2** show a theoretic model that could help to understand the pathway from diabetes to disability.[32]

Obesity and cardiovascular disease were factors explaining most of the excess odds of disability associated with diabetes.[24,26] There seems that the association between diabetes and disability is independent of BMI. In WHAS, adjustment for BMI did not change the relationships of diabetes and any of the disability groups,[24] and slightly reduced the association between diabetes and objective measures of physical function.[21]

Cardiovascular disease is a major cause of disability[33] and people with diabetes have greater risk of developing cardiovascular disease. In NHANES, coronary heart disease (CHD) and stroke were the main contributing risk factors of diabetes-related disability. In men, the risk was 25% and 21%, respectively. In women, the risk of excess disability was 34% for CHD and 14% for stroke.[26] Stroke history among

Impairment	**Functional Limitation**	**Disability**
Anatomical, physiological, mental or emotional abnormalities or loss	Limitation in performance at the level of the whole organism or person	Limitation in performance of socially defined roles and tasks within a sociocultural and physical environment

Distinctions

Both **impairment** and **functional limitation** involve function

Impairment – reference is to the levels of tissues, organs and systems
Functional limitation - reference is to the level of the person as a whole

Functional limitation refers to organismic performance; **disability** refers to social performance

Disability is a relational concept, whereas the other three stages (pathology, impairment, functional limitation) are concepts of attributes

Fig. 1. Differentiating functional limitation from impairment and disability. (*Modified from Nagi SZ. An epidemiology of disability among adults in the United States. Milbank Mem Fund Q Health Soc 1976;54:439–67.*)

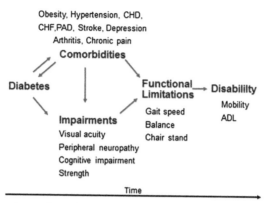

Fig. 2. Theoretic pathway from diabetes to disability. CHD, coronary heart disease; CHF, congestive heart failure; PAD, peripheral arterial disease. (*Adapted from* Volpato S, Maraldi C, Fellin R. Type 2 diabetes and risk for functional decline and disability in older persons. Curr Diabetes Rev 2010;6:134–43.)

the diabetic population significantly increased the risk of developing mobility impairment by 123% and the risk of ADL disability by 92%.[34]

Lower-extremity diseases, including peripheral arterial disease (PAD) and peripheral nerve dysfunction (PND), are important disabling diabetes complications that could contribute to this excess disability burden. Controlling for PAD decreased the excess risk of mobility disability associated with diabetes by 30% in WHAS.[35] PND was significantly associated with poorer lower-extremity physical performance[36] but explained only a portion of the association of diabetes with physical disability.[37] The effect of diabetes on lower-extremity function was decreased by 19% after adjustment for neuropathy measures, suggesting that PND partially mediates the relationship between diabetes and physical function.[38]

Older adults with type 2 diabetes have twice the likelihood of developing cognitive impairment and dementia.[39] The underlying pathophysiological mechanisms are multifactorial, including those common to both Alzheimer's disease and vascular dementia. Cognitive impairment and dementia are strong predictors of declines in gait speed[40] and poorer SPPB.[41]

Depression is another associated diabetes comorbidity that contributes to ADL and mobility disability.[42] Prevalence of depressive symptoms is higher in people with diabetes than in their nondiabetic counterparts.[43] Diabetes is a risk factor for incident depression,[44] with a high risk among those having poor glycemic control.[45] In WHAS, depression was one of the main factors contributing to 24% of the excessive disability risk.[35] Evaluation of the presence of depressive symptoms in older adults with diabetes is crucial because depression is associated with risk of poor diabetes management and poor adherence to treatment leading to poor glycemic control and risk of developing diabetes complications.

Poor glycemic control and long duration of diabetes increase the risk of developing diabetic complications. Glycemic control assessed by the HbA1C level and comorbidities explained up to 85% of the excess odds of disability but poor glycemic control (HbA1C ≥8%) alone only accounted for up to 10% of these excess odds.[25] Higher HbA1c (HbA1c 8.0%–8.9%) was associated with less functional decline at 2 years in community-dwelling, nursing home–eligible individuals with diabetes.[46] In contrast, others found that poor glycemic control (HbA1c ≥7%) contributes to the relationship between diabetes and functional limitation in a well-functioning older population.[18] In Mexican-American and European American older adults with diabetes, short-term and long-term maintenance of lower-extremity function over a 36-month period were both greater in the better glycemic control group (HbA1c <7%) than in the poorer control group.[47] Longer diabetes duration has been shown to be associated with mobility disability in both men and women.[25,26] However, other studies did not find any relationship between duration of diabetes and disability in older adults with diabetes.[18,27]

Older adults with diabetes had increased levels of inflammatory markers.[48] Increased levels of these markers were also associated with ADL and mobility disability.[49] Among participants with diabetes in a well-functioning study population, those with higher inflammatory markers had an increased risk of functional decline, suggesting that inflammation was an independent risk of disability among those with diabetes.[50]

Prevalence of chronic pain is high in older persons, reported by almost 55% of those with diabetes,[51] and is strongly associated with physical function.[52] PND, PAD, foot ulcers, arthritis, and other causes of musculoskeletal pain are common potential causes of pain in older patients with diabetes. In WHAS, pain was a cause of progression of mobility disability.[53]

Insulin resistance (IR) is a key pathophysiological determinant of type 2 diabetes. No study to date has evaluated the role of IR as a potential mediator but, among older adults without diabetes, IR has been found associated with poorer gait speed.[54]

Diabetes is associated with a higher risk of falls.[55] See the article by Vinik and colleagues elsewhere in this issue for further exploration of this topic.

Higher prevalence of cardiovascular disease, peripheral neuropathy, poor balance, orthostatic hypotension, visual impairment, cognitive impairment, pain, and obesity might contribute to the increased risk of falls in this population.[56] Most of these diabetes complications are potentially prevented or delayed by optimal glycemic control, though the use of insulin therapy or intensive glycemic control may also be related to the risk of falls in older adults with diabetes.[57,58]

Although all these diabetes complications and diabetes-associated comorbidities accounted for the excess risk of disability (1) in most of the studies no single condition could explain this association and (2) even after adjustment for all these comorbidities, diabetes was still associated with excessive disability burden,[18,25,26,32] suggesting that other factors could explain this relationship. Because some of these diabetes-related comorbidities are potential modifiable risk factors of disability (**Table 2**), preventing and reducing the excess risk of disability associated with diabetes might be possible but this needs to be further studied in clinical trials.

MUSCLE STRENGTH AND MUSCLE QUALITY

Recent clinical and epidemiologic studies have suggested an accelerated loss of muscle mass and muscle strength as additional potential mediators of the association between diabetes and disability.[59] The progressive loss of muscle mass and strength, often referred to as sarcopenia, increases the difficulty during ADL and, as consequence, strongly increases the risk of functional dependency.[60] Although strongly related to the aging process, sarcopenia is a multifactorial process in which multiple conditions, including genetic characteristics, life-style factors, hormonal and metabolic status, and several chronic diseases, play as causal factors.[61]

Regardless the total amount of muscle mass, however, older diabetic individuals have been consistently characterized by lower muscle strength in different body segments. Most of the studies that addressed this topic were designed to investigate the

Table 2	
Risk factors for disability in older adults with diabetes	
Nonmodifiable	**Potentially Modifiable**
• Age • Duration of diabetes • Genetic background	Diabetes-related comorbidities • Peripheral neuropathies • CHD • PAD • Visual impairment • Congestive heart failure • Stroke • Poor glycemic control Diabetes-associated comorbidities • Obesity • Cognitive impairment or dementia • Depressive symptoms • Arthritis • Widespread and lower-extremity pain Other • Sarcopenia • Poor muscle quality • Low-grade systemic inflammation • Oxidative stress

Abbreviations: CHD, coronary heart disease; PAD, peripheral arterial disease.
Data from Volpato S, Maraldi C, Fellin R. Type 2 diabetes and risk for functional decline and disability in older persons. Curr Diabetes Rev 2010;6:134–43.

relationship between type 2 diabetes and mobility or ADL disability, and only a few specifically investigated the association between diabetes and strength of the upper extremities, with controversial results. Multiple well-known population-based cohort studies have investigated the link between diabetes and muscle function in older persons (**Table 3**).[62–65] In cross-sectional analyse, all the studies reported a significant and independent association between diabetes and leg muscle strength.[19] Furthermore, a longitudinal analysis from the Health, Aging, and Body Composition (Health ABC) study demonstrated that older men and women with diabetes had a steeper strength decline over time compared with nondiabetic persons.[62] These results support the hypothesis of a causal link between diabetes and reduced skeletal muscle strength.

Results from recent epidemiologic and clinical studies suggest that older people with diabetes, despite having adequate skeletal muscle mass, tended to have reduced skeletal muscle strength and muscle performance, and a more rapid decline in muscle mass and lower extremity strength over time. Several investigators hypothesize that the detrimental effect of dysglycemia and other diabetes-related metabolic abnormalities on skeletal muscle would be better captured by qualitative measures rather than quantitative indicators of muscle mass. Although strongly correlated with muscle function, several studies have consistently demonstrated that muscle mass explains less than 50% of muscle strength variability.[66] The term muscle quality is, therefore, used to define a composite measure of muscle strength standardized for an indicator of muscle mass.

In the InCHIANTI (Invecchiare in Chianti) study, in which muscle quality was defined as the ratio of lower limb muscle strength over calf muscle area, participants with

Table 3
Major epidemiologic studies investigating skeletal muscle strength, according to diabetes status

Study	N Follow-Up	Gender	Skeletal Muscle Groups	Significant Association	Statistical Adjustment
Cross-sectional studies					
Health ABC[63]	2618	Men/Women	Knee: extension Hand: grip strength	Yes Yes in men; No in women	Age, race, education, smoking, drinking, body mass index, physical activity, comorbidity
InCHIANTI[21]	835	Men/Women	Hip: abduction or adduction Hip: flexion or extension Knee: extension or flexion Ankle: dorsoplantar flexion	Yes	Age, gender
NHANES1999–02[19]	2573	Men/Women	Knee: extension	Yes	Demographics, weight, height, physical activity, CRP
Hertfordshire Cohort Study[64]	1391	Men/Women	Hand: grip strength	Yes	Body weight
SOF[65]	2864	Women	Hand: grip strength	No	None
Prospective studies					
HEALTH ABC[62]	1840, 3 y	Men/Women	Knee: extension	Yes	Age, gender, race, education, smoking, drinking, body mass index, physical activity, comorbidity
SOF[65]	2864, 4.9 y	Women	Grip strength	No	Age, race, clinic site, baseline physical performance measure, body mass index, self-rated health, hypertension, and estrogen use

Abbreviations: CRP, C-reactive protein; Health ABC, Health, Aging and Body Composition study; InCHIANTI, Invecchiare in Chianti; NHANES, National Health and Nutrition Examination Surveys; SOF, Study of Osteoporotic Fractures.

diabetes, despite having a greater skeletal muscle calf area, had poorer muscle quality and lower muscle power. In the multivariate regression models, lower-limb muscle characteristics accounted for 24.3% and 15.1% of walking speed difference between diabetic and nondiabetic subjects in the 4-m and 400-m walks, respectively.[21]

There are multiple potential biological pathways for explaining why older adults with diabetes tend to have greater decline of skeletal muscle strength and performance. First, in patients with long-standing disease, the presence of classic diabetes complications includes peripheral neuropathy and obstructive arterial disease, 2 powerful risk factors for sarcopenia and gait impairment.[67,68] Second, insulin plays a key role in protein anabolism; indeed, amino acids and insulin have a synergistic effect on stimulating muscle protein anabolism.[69,70] It has also been shown that insulin deficiency leads to a protein catabolic state with loss of muscle mass that could be reversed by insulin therapy. Furthermore, hyperglycemia is associated with multiple metabolic abnormalities potentially correlated with muscle cell damage, including plasma-free fatty acid and proinflammatory cytokines concentrations elevation. It has been hypothesized that an intramuscular inflammation-related pathway can induce a proteolytic process in skeletal muscle.[71] Increased muscle fat infiltration, which results in a loss of muscle quality and in decreased muscle density, has been associated with both reduced oxidative activity and maximal aerobic capacity. Furthermore, in epidemiologic studies of older persons, fat infiltration predicted the risk of mobility disability over time.[72]

SUMMARY

Results from cross-sectional and longitudinal observational studies showed that older adults with diabetes are at increased risk of functional limitation and ADL, IADL, and mobility disability.[1,22,24–31] Although several impairments or comorbidities, related or not to diabetes, could account for this excessive disability risk, no single condition could explain the association of diabetes with disability.[18,25,26,32] Greater decline in muscle strength and poorer muscle quality observed in older adults with diabetes compared with their nondiabetic counterparts could also be potential mediators of the association between diabetes and disability.[21,59] As some diabetes-related or diabetes-associated comorbidities are potential modifiable risk factors for disability in older adults with diabetes, prevention or reduction of the excessive risk of disability associated with diabetes might be feasible. Clinical trials focusing on reducing the onset of these diabetes-related or diabetes-associated comorbidities are needed to examine their potential impact in slowing the decline in physical function in older adults with diabetes.

REFERENCES

1. Guralnik JM, LaCroix AZ, Abbott RD, et al. Maintaining mobility in late life. I. Demographic characteristics and chronic conditions. Am J Epidemiol 1993;137: 845–57.
2. Seeman TE, Merkin SS, Crimmins EM, et al. Disability trends among older Americans: national health and nutrition examination surveys, 1988–1994 and 1999–2004. Am J Public Health 2010;100:100–7.
3. Fried LP, Guralnik JM. Disability in older adults: evidence regarding significance, etiology, and risk. J Am Geriatr Soc 1997;45:92–100.
4. Boyle JP, Honeycutt AA, Narayan KM, et al. Projection of diabetes burden through 2050: impact of changing demography and disease prevalence in the U.S. Diabetes Care 2001;24:1936–40.

5. Volpato S, Maraldi C. Diabetes and disability, cognitive decline, and aging-related outcomes. In: Narayan KM, Gregg EW, Cowie CC, et al, editors. Diabetes public health: from research to policy. Oxford (United Kingdom): Oxford University Press; 2010. p. 225–45.

6. Wong EB, Gearon E, Harding J, et al. Diabetes and risk of physical disability in adults: a systematic review and meta-analysis. Lancet Diabetes Endocrinol 2013;1:106–14.

7. Nagi SZ. An epidemiology of disability among adults in the United States. Milbank Mem Fund Q Health Soc 1976;54:439–67.

8. Guralnik JM, Ferrucci L, Simonsick EM, et al. Lower-extremity function in persons over the age of 70 years as a predictor of subsequent disability. N Engl J Med 1995;332:556–61.

9. Penninx BW, Ferrucci L, Leveille SG, et al. Lower extremity performance in nondisabled older persons as a predictor of subsequent hospitalization. J Gerontol A Biol Sci Med Sci 2000;55:M691–7.

10. Studenski S, Perera S, Wallace D, et al. Physical performance measures in the clinical setting. J Am Geriatr Soc 2003;51:314–22.

11. Guralnik JM, Simonsick EM, Ferrucci L, et al. A short physical performance battery assessing lower extremity function: association with self-reported disability and prediction of mortality and nursing home placement. J Gerontol 1994;49:M85–94.

12. Lawton MP, Brody EM. Assessment of older people: self-maintaining and instrumental activities of daily living. Gerontologist 1969;9:179–86.

13. Branch LG, Jette AM. A prospective study of long-term care institutionalization among the aged. Am J Public Health 1982;72:1373–9.

14. Bharucha AJ, Pandav R, Shen C, et al. Predictors of nursing facility admission: a 12-year epidemiological study in the United States. J Am Geriatr Soc 2004;52: 434–9.

15. Keller BK, Potter JF. Predictors of mortality in outpatient geriatric evaluation and management clinic patients. J Gerontol 1994;49:M246–51.

16. Hardy SE, Kang Y, Studenski SA, et al. Ability to walk 1/4 mile predicts subsequent disability, mortality, and health care costs. J Gen Intern Med 2011;26:130–5.

17. Ferrucci L, Penninx BW, Leveille SG, et al. Characteristics of nondisabled older persons who perform poorly in objective tests of lower extremity function. J Am Geriatr Soc 2000;48:1102–10.

18. de Rekeneire N, Resnick HE, Schwartz AV, et al. Diabetes is associated with subclinical functional limitation in nondisabled older individuals: the Health, Aging, and Body Composition study. Diabetes Care 2003;26:3257–63.

19. Kalyani RR, Tra Y, Yeh HC, et al. Quadriceps strength, quadriceps power, and gait speed in older U.S. adults with diabetes mellitus: results from the national health and nutrition examination survey, 1999-2002. J Am Geriatr Soc 2013; 61:769–75.

20. Ko SU, Stenholm S, Chia CW, et al. Gait pattern alterations in older adults associated with type 2 diabetes in the absence of peripheral neuropathy—results from the Baltimore Longitudinal Study of Aging. Gait Posture 2011;34:548–52.

21. Volpato S, Bianchi L, Lauretani F, et al. Role of muscle mass and muscle quality in the association between diabetes and gait speed. Diabetes Care 2012;35: 1672–9.

22. Volpato S, Ferrucci L, Blaum C, et al. Progression of lower-extremity disability in older women with diabetes: the Women's Health and Aging Study. Diabetes Care 2003;26:0–5.

23. Onder G, Penninx BW, Ferrucci L, et al. Measures of physical performance and risk for progressive and catastrophic disability: results from the Women's Health and Aging Study. J Gerontol A Biol Sci Med Sci 2005;60A:74–9.
24. Maty SC, Fried LP, Volpato S, et al. Patterns of disability related to diabetes mellitus in older women. J Gerontol A Biol Sci Med Sci 2004;59:148–53.
25. Kalyani RR, Saudek CD, Brancati FL, et al. Association of diabetes, comorbidities, and A1C with functional disability in older adults: results from the national health and nutrition examination survey (NHANES), 1999-2006. Diabetes Care 2010;33:1055–60.
26. Gregg EW, Beckles GL, Williamson DF, et al. Diabetes and physical disability among older U.S. adults. Diabetes Care 2000;23:1272–7.
27. Gregg EW, Mangione CM, Cauley JA, et al, Study of Osteoporotic Fractures Research Group. Diabetes and incidence of functional disability in older women. Diabetes Care 2002;25:61–7.
28. Bourdel-Marchasson I, Dubroca B, Manciet G, et al. Prevalence of diabetes and effect on quality of life in older French living in the community: the PAQUID epidemiological survey. J Am Geriatr Soc 1997;45:295–301.
29. Maggi S, Noale M, Gallina P, et al, ILSA Group. Physical disability among older Italians with diabetes. The ILSA study. Diabetologia 2004;47:1957–62.
30. Chau PH, Woo J, Lee CH, et al. Older people with diabetes have higher risk of depression, cognitive and functional impairments: implications for diabetes services. J Nutr Health Aging 2011;15:751–5.
31. Guccione AA, Felson DT, Anderson JJ, et al. The effects of specific medical conditions on the functional limitations of elders in the Framingham study. Am J Public Health 1994;84:351–8.
32. Volpato S, Maraldi C, Fellin R. Type 2 diabetes and risk for functional decline and disability in older persons. Curr Diabetes Rev 2010;6:134–43.
33. Pinsky JL, Jette AM, Branch LG, et al. The Framingham Disability Study: relationship of various coronary heart disease manifestations to disability in older persons living in the community. Am J Public Health 1990;80:1363–7.
34. Bruce DG, Davis WA, Davis TME. Longitudinal predictors of reduced mobility and physical disability in patients with type 2 diabetes: the Fremantle Diabetes Study. Diabetes Care 2005;28:2441–7.
35. Volpato S, Blaum C, Resnick H, et al, Women's Health and Aging Study. Comorbidities and impairments explaining the association between diabetes and lower extremity disability: the Women's Health and Aging Study. Diabetes Care 2002;25:678–83.
36. Resnick HE, Vinik AI, Schwartz AV, et al. Independent effects of peripheral nerve dysfunction on lower-extremity physical function in old age: the Women's Health and Aging Study. Diabetes Care 2000;23:1642–7.
37. Strotmeyer E, de Rekeneire N, Schwartz A, et al. The relationship of reduced peripheral nerve function and diabetes with physical performance in older white and black adults: the Health, Aging, and Body Composition (Health ABC) study. Diabetes Care 2008;31:1767–72.
38. Chiles NS, Phillips CL, Volpato S, et al. Diabetes, peripheral neuropathy, and lower-extremity function. J Gen Intern Med 2014;28:91–5.
39. Biessels GJ, Staekenborg S, Brunner E, et al. Risk of dementia in diabetes mellitus: a systematic review. Lancet Neurol 2006;5:64–74.
40. Atkinson HH, Cesari M, Kritchevsky SB, et al. Predictors of combined cognitive and physical decline. J Am Geriatr Soc 2005;53:1197–202.

41. Bruce-Keller AJ, Brouillette RM, Tudor-Locke C, et al. Relationship between cognitive domains, physical performance, and gait in elderly and demented subjects. J Alzheimers Dis 2012;30:899–908.

42. Penninx BW, Leveille S, Ferrucci L, et al. Exploring the effect of depression on physical disability: longitudinal evidence from the established populations for epidemiologic studies of the elderly. Am J Public Health 1999;89:1346–52.

43. Anderson RJ, Freedland KE, Clouse RE, et al. The prevalence of comorbid depression in adults with diabetes: a meta-analysis. Diabetes Care 2001;24:1069–78.

44. Rotella F, Mannucci E. Diabetes mellitus as a risk factor for depression. A meta-analysis of longitudinal studies. Diabetes Res Clin Pract 2013;99:98–104.

45. Maraldi C, Volpato S, Penninx BW, et al. Diabetes mellitus, glycemic control, and incident depressive symptoms among 70- to 79-year-old persons; the health, aging, and body composition study. Arch Intern Med 2007;167:1137–44.

46. Yau CK, Eng C, Cenzer IS, et al. Glycosylated hemoglobin and functional decline in community-dwelling nursing home-eligible elderly adults with diabetes mellitus. J Am Geriatr Soc 2012;60:1215–21.

47. Wang CP, Hazuda HP. Better glycemic control is associated with maintenance of lower-extremity function over time in Mexican American and European American older adults with diabetes. Diabetes Care 2011;34:268–73.

48. Barzilay JI, Abraham L, Heckbert SR, et al. The relation of markers of inflammation to the development of glucose disorders in the elderly: the Cardiovascular Health Study. Diabetes 2001;50:2384–9.

49. Penninx BW, Kritchevsky SB, Newman AB, et al. Inflammatory markers and incident mobility limitation in the elderly. J Am Geriatr Soc 2004;52:1105–13.

50. Figaro MK, Kritchevsky SB, Resnick HE, et al. Diabetes, inflammation, and functional decline in older adults: findings from the Health, Aging and Body Composition (ABC) study. Diabetes Care 2006;29:2039–45.

51. Krein SL, Heisler M, Piette JD, et al. The effect of chronic pain on diabetes patients' self-management. Diabetes Care 2005;28:65–70.

52. Patel KV, Guralnik JM, Dansie EJ, et al. Prevalence and impact of pain among older adults in the United States: findings from the 2011 National Health and Aging Trends Study. Pain 2013;154:2649–57.

53. Leveille SG, Guralnik JM, Hochberg M, et al. Low back pain and disability in older women: independent association with difficulty but not inability to perform daily activities. J Gerontol A Biol Sci Med Sci 1999;54:M487–93.

54. Kuo CK, Lin LY, Yu YH, et al. Inverse association between insulin resistance and gait speed in nondiabetic older men: results from the U.S. national health and nutrition examination survey (NHANES) 1999-2002. BMC Geriatr 2009;9:49.

55. Schwartz AV, Hillier TA, Sellmeyer DE, et al. Older women with diabetes have a higher risk of falls: a prospective study. Diabetes Care 2002;25:1749–54.

56. Volpato S, Leveille SG, Blaum C, et al. Risk factors for falls in older disabled women with diabetes: the Women's Health and Aging Study. J Gerontol A Biol Sci Med Sci 2005;60:1539–45.

57. Huang ES, Karter AJ, Danielson KK, et al. The association between the number of prescription medications and incident falls in a multi-ethnic population of adult type-2 diabetes patients: the diabetes and aging study. J Gen Intern Med 2010;25:141–6.

58. Schwartz AV, Vittinghoff E, Sellmeyer DE, et al. Diabetes-related complications, glycemic control, and falls in older adults. Diabetes Care 2008;31:391–6.

59. Landi F, Onder G, Bernabei R. Sarcopenia and diabetes: two sides of the same coin. J Am Med Dir Assoc 2013;14:540–1.

60. Rosenberg IH. Sarcopenia: origins and clinical relevance. J Nutr 1997;127: 990–1.

61. Volpato S, Bianchi L, Cherubini A, et al. Prevalence and clinical correlates of sarcopenia in community-dwelling older people: application of the EWGSOP definition and diagnostic algorithm. J Gerontol A Biol Sci Med Sci 2014;69(4): 438–46.

62. Park SW, Goodpaster BH, Strotmeyer ES, et al. Accelerated loss of skeletal muscle strength in older adults with type 2 diabetes. The health, aging, and body composition study. Diabetes Care 2007;30:1507–12.

63. Park SW, Goodpaster BH, Strotmeyer ES, et al. Decreased muscle strength and quality in older adults with type 2 diabetes: the health, aging, and body composition study. Diabetes 2006;55:1813–8.

64. Sayer AA, Dennison EM, Syddall HE, et al. Type 2 diabetes, muscle strength, and impaired physical function: the tip of the iceberg? Diabetes Care 2005; 28:2541–2.

65. Lee CG, Schwartz AV, Yaffe K, et al. Changes in physical performance in older women according to presence and treatment of diabetes mellitus. J Am Geriatr Soc 2013;61:1872–8.

66. Manini TM, Clark BC. Dynapenia and aging: an update. J Gerontol A Biol Sci Med Sci 2012;67:28–40.

67. Martinelli AR, Mantovani AM, Nozabieli AJ, et al. Muscle strength and ankle mobility for the gait parameters in diabetic neuropathies. Foot (Edinb) 2013; 23:317–21.

68. McDermott MM, Guralnik JM, Albay M, et al. Impairments of muscles and nerves associated with peripheral arterial disease and their relationship with lower extremity functioning: the InCHIANTI study. J Am Geriatr Soc 2004;52: 405–10.

69. Wolfe RR. Effects of insulin on muscle tissue. Curr Opin Clin Nutr Metab Care 2000;3:67–71.

70. Bassil MS, Gougeon R. Muscle protein anabolism in type 2 diabetes. Curr Opin Clin Nutr Metab Care 2013;16:83–8.

71. Lee SW, Dai G, Hu Z, et al. Regulation of muscle protein degradation: coordinated control of apoptotic and ubiquitin-proteasome systems by phosphatidylinositol 3 kinase. J Am Soc Nephrol 2004;15:1537–45.

72. Visser M, Goodpaster BH, Kritchevsky SB, et al. Muscle mass, muscle strength, and muscle fat infiltration as predictors of incident mobility limitations in well-functioning older persons. J Gerontol A Biol Sci Med Sci 2005;60:324–33.

Links Between Osteoarthritis and Diabetes

Implications for Management from a Physical Activity Perspective

Sara R. Piva, PhD, PT, OCS[a,*], Allyn M. Susko, PT, DPT[a],
Samannaaz S. Khoja, PT, MS[a], Deborah A. Josbeno, PhD, PT, NCS[a],
G. Kelley Fitzgerald, PhD, PT[a], Frederico G.S. Toledo, MD[b]

KEYWORDS

- Type 2 diabetes • Osteoarthritis • Risk factors • Glucose metabolism • Arthritis
- Physical activity • Exercise

KEY POINTS

- Individuals with type 2 diabetes mellitus (T2DM) are more susceptible to developing osteoarthritis (OA), partially because these conditions share etiologic factors, including aging and obesity.
- Aging- and obesity-related physical and physiologic impairments contribute to the development of OA (eg, muscle weakness/atrophy, poor balance, deconditioning, pain, excess joint loads, abnormal lipid metabolism, low-grade inflammation, and oxidative stress).
- Hyperglycemia may also directly injure cartilage health in OA by mechanisms involving advanced glycation end-products (AGEs) and peripheral neuropathy.
- Physical activity is the only available intervention capable of positively affecting the impairments that link aging, OA, and T2DM.
- Special considerations are necessary for safe and effective implementation of physical activity programs in older adults with OA and T2DM.

INTRODUCTION

Osteoarthritis (OA) and type 2 diabetes mellitus (T2DM) are 2 prevalent chronic diseases in the United States. OA affects 14% of adults aged 25 years and older

[a] Department of Physical Therapy, School of Health and Rehabilitation Sciences, University of Pittsburgh, Bridgeside Point 1, 100 Technology Drive, Suite 210, Pittsburgh, PA 15219, USA; [b] Division of Endocrinology and Metabolism, Department of Medicine, University of Pittsburgh, 200 Lothrop Street, BST E1140, Pittsburgh, PA 15261, USA
* Corresponding author.
E-mail address: spiva@pitt.edu

Clin Geriatr Med 31 (2015) 67–87
http://dx.doi.org/10.1016/j.cger.2014.08.019
0749-0690/15/$ – see front matter © 2015 Elsevier Inc. All rights reserved.

and 34% of those over the age of 65.[1] OA is a leading cause of disability and economic burden; around 40% of adults with OA report arthritis-related limitations in daily activities and 30% report difficulties in work-related tasks.[1] Diabetes affects 12% of adults 20 years and older and 26% of those over the age of 65.[2] Diabetes is associated with mortality and serious complications, such as heart disease, stroke, kidney failure, and lower limb amputation.[2]

In the aging population, the coexistence of OA and T2DM is frequent and can be a source of greater disability and economic burden.[3,4] There seems to be an increased susceptibility to develop OA in those with T2DM.[5,6] A recent report in adults ranging from 18 to 64 years showed that the prevalence of arthritis was 52% in those with T2DM compared with 27% in those without T2DM.[7] The reason for the high prevalence of arthritis in those with T2DM is not entirely clear. OA and T2DM share common risk factors, such as obesity and advanced aging, which may explain the higher prevalence of OA in the diabetic population.[8] More recently, OA has been associated with systemic metabolic disturbances commonly seen in T2DM, suggesting that diabetes in and of itself influences the pathophysiology of OA independently of obesity or aging per se. These metabolic alterations have been proposed to serve as an underlying link between OA and T2DM.

With the growing prevalence of older persons diagnosed with both OA and T2DM, adequate prevention and management of these combined conditions becomes necessary. Optimal care of these patients depends on understanding the risk factors leading to the development and progression of these commonly coexisting conditions. The purpose of this paper is to review the evidence on common risk factors and to discuss emerging underlying links between OA and T2DM. The review also discusses treatment considerations from a physical activity perspective when older individuals have both OA and T2DM.

SHARED RISK FACTORS FOR OSTEOARTHRITIS AND TYPE 2 DIABETES MELLITUS
Age and Obesity

Demographic and physiologic risk factors for OA and T2DM are listed in **Table 1**. It is not surprising that OA and T2DM coexist; they share several common risk factors, with age being a recognized link. The increased risk for OA and T2DM with aging is multifactorial. One factor is the decline in cell function with aging. For example, aging is associated with T2DM in part because pancreatic β-cell function declines with aging.[9] Aging also causes OA. In OA, senescent chondrocytes are more likely than young chondrocytes to secrete inflammatory mediators involved in cartilage degradation.[10] Living longer also promotes cumulative joint loads and consequent cartilage wear and OA. Finally, aging has been attributed to a decline in mitochondrial health, and decreased mitochondrial health has been theorized to contribute to both diabetes and cartilage degradation.[11–15]

Obesity is exceedingly prevalent among individuals with T2DM, and participates in the pathogenesis of T2DM. Obesity is also a risk factor for OA. Obesity contributes to the development of OA via biomechanical and systemic pathways. The biomechanical pathway is based on the direct effects of increased body weight. For example, increased body weight imposes greater loads on the weight-bearing joints, which has been shown to affect cartilage wear.[16,17] Excess body weight has also been associated with misalignment of weight-bearing joints (particularly the knee joint), which increases joint stress and promotes cartilage degradation that lead to OA.[18] Moreover, obesity has been linked with decreased strength in muscles necessary for joint stabilization and therefore decreased ability to sustain mechanical joint stress.[19,20]

Table 1
Risk factors for osteoarthritis (OA) and diabetes

Risk Factors for OA	Risk Factors for Diabetes
Female sex	High-risk ethnic or racial group (African
History of joint injury	American, Latino, Native American, Asian
Osteoporosis/reduced bone mineral density	American, Pacific Islander)
Occupational or repetitive joint stress	Family history of diabetes
	History of gestational diabetes or giving
	birth to an infant >9 pounds
	Sedentary lifestyle

Risk Factors Common for OA and Diabetes	
Age	Age
Overweight or obese (body mass index >25)	Overweight or obese (body mass index >25)
Hypertension[a]	Hypertension
Dyslipidemia[a]	Dyslipidemia (low high-density lipoprotein
Impaired glucose tolerance[a]	and/or high triglyceride)
	Impaired glucose tolerance (prediabetes)

[a] Risk factors that need further validation.
Data from Refs.[102–104]

Although physical joint stress may be an important factor for obesity-mediated OA, it does not seem to be the only factor. An increased risk for OA in non–weight-bearing joints, such as those of the hands, has been previously reported in obesity,[21] suggesting there is a systemic, nonmechanical influence on the risk for OA. This systemic link is not well understood, but there are theoretic precedents for supporting such notion. Obesity causes chronic low-grade inflammation in adipose tissue and enhanced expression and secretion of proinflammatory cytokines (eg, interleukin [IL]-6, IL-1, and tumor necrosis factor-α) as well as adipokines (eg, leptin, adiponectin, resistin, and visfatin).[15,22] IL-1 and tumor necrosis factor-α have been shown to mediate the OA pathophysiology, possibly by modulating chondrocyte expression of proteases involved in matrix breakdown.

Adipokines are active in cartilage regulation and have been linked to the development of OA.[23] Specifically, studies have shown that leptin is present in synovial fluid of joints with OA and high levels of this hormone in the synovial fluid are strongly associated with the radiographic severity of OA.[24,25] High plasma levels of leptin are seen in obesity, but it is unclear whether the association between leptin and OA severity is merely a coincidence or reflects an underlying pathophysiologic link. Adiponectin is another adipokine, but its role in OA has been conflicting. One study reported higher levels of adiponectin in patients with erosive OA compared with those with nonerosive OA,[26] whereas another study demonstrated that increased levels of this molecule protect against the progression of hand OA.[27] For a comprehensive review on the role of adipokines to OA see the review from Conde and colleagues.[28]

Hypertension and Dyslipidemia

Hypertension and dyslipidemia, both widely recognized risk factors for T2DM,[29,30] have been proposed to contribute to the development of OA.[31–33] It has been theorized that hypertension might affect OA via narrowing of blood vessels and subchondral ischemia, which would initiate cartilage degradation.[33,34] Although several studies demonstrated higher prevalence of OA in individuals with hypertension,[35–38] adjustments for obesity were not conducted in those studies; therefore, the contribution of hypertension to OA needs further investigation.

Evidence for the contribution of dyslipidemia in OA is also not conclusive (for a comprehensive review of this topic, see papers from Velasquez and colleagues[32] and Zhuo and associates[33]). One study demonstrated a positive association between serum cholesterol levels and OA independent of obesity. Others have demonstrated that patients with OA have increased lipid deposits in the chondrocytes and deregulation of cellular lipid metabolism that might initiate OA development.[31] There is also evidence that fatty acids are elevated in OA bone and that excessive intake of polyunsaturated fatty acids is associated with increased risk of bone marrow lesions.[39–44] However, it is important to make a distinction between circulating lipid levels and lipid metabolism within tissues, which should not be equated to each other and follow different metabolic regulation. These studies should be interpreted as hypothesis-generating because they do not definitely demonstrate that dyslipidemia is an etiologic factor in OA.

Among the common risk factors for OA and T2DM, aging and obesity have a major impact on the functional ability in these individuals. Aging is characterized by physiologic changes such as altered endocrine function, loss of skeletal muscle function (decreased lean mass and muscle strength), and poor balance, as well as lifestyle changes such as decreased physical activity and nutritional deficiencies; all of these factors contribute to declines in functional ability and overall health.[45] Studies have also shown that obese people demonstrate an increased incidence of pain in the weight-bearing joints and a higher pain perception during activity.[46–48] The increased pain is likely mediated by heightened systemic inflammation and has been shown to be strongly related to the degree of disability in obese individuals.[49] Thus, obesity-related factors such as increased pain, muscle weakness, and joint misalignment also limit mobility and contribute to functional limitations.

ASSOCIATION BETWEEN OSTEOARTHRITIS AND TYPE 2 DIABETES MELLITUS
Does Type 2 Diabetes Mellitus Independently Contribute to Osteoarthritis?

Because OA and T2DM share common risk factors, the independent contribution of T2DM on OA is difficult to study. Several studies have tried to answer the question of whether T2DM predicts OA independently of age and obesity. Earlier studies failed to report significant associations.[6,50,51] However, these studies had methodological limitations, such as (1) the selection of fairly subjective criteria for the diagnosis of OA,[50] (2) having subjects with knee OA grouped by diabetes status but poorly matched for weight,[51] (3) assessment of generalized OA based only on radiographs of either hands and hips or hands and knees,[6] or (4) small sample sizes.[6,51] Therefore, conclusions from those studies are far from definitive and should be approached with caution.

Nonetheless, recent studies have demonstrated an independent association between T2DM status and OA.[5,52] Results of a 20-year longitudinal cohort study of 927 individuals suggest that T2DM predicts both joint failure and hip and knee arthroplasty surgery, independently of age, sex, and body mass index.[5] This study used both clinical measures (Knee Injury and Osteoarthritis Outcome Score, Western Ontario and McMaster Universities Osteoarthritis Index) and advanced imaging techniques (ultrasonography) to assess the severity of OA. In support of these findings, another study reported that individuals with T2DM had increased odds for clinical diagnosis of knee and hand OA (consistent with American College of Rheumatology criteria) after adjusting for age and body mass index.[52] Because these recent studies have used better methodologic approaches and designs, stronger evidence is accumulating in favor of an independent contribution of T2DM to the development and progression of OA.

Potential Underlying Links Between Osteoarthritis and Type 2 Diabetes Mellitus

Cartilage health depends on a number of metabolic processes that regulate cartilage growth and nutrition that, if altered, can lead to its degradation.[53] Several investigators have postulated that altered glucose metabolism could be a direct link between OA and T2DM.[10,21,32,54,55] Rosa and colleagues[54] investigated how glucose concentrations affect chondrocyte function in vitro using cartilage samples from healthy donors (posthumously) and from patients with OA undergoing total knee arthroplasty. The cartilage samples were treated with varying concentrations of glucose in the medium and cartilage function measured. Findings revealed that chondrocytes of those with OA were unable to downregulate glucose transport into the chondrocyte in a hyperglycemic environment compared with a normoglycemic one. Higher levels of reactive oxygen species were also detected in OA cartilage treated in a hyperglycemic-like environment, unlike the reactive oxygen species levels in normal chondrocytes treated with high glucose medium. Reactive oxygen species are harmful to chondrocytes because they favor production of cytokines, such as IL-1β, and transcription factors, such as nuclear factor-κB, which give rise to catabolic processes implicated in cell degradation and cell apoptosis.[56] The same group conducted a similar study to measure the effect of glucose concentrations on expression of proteolytic enzymes, mainly matrix metalloproteases, which are responsible for cartilage degradation. Findings revealed a higher trend in the expression of matrix metalloproteases in OA chondrocytes treated with hyperglycemic medium compared with normal chondrocytes in a hyperglycemic medium.[57] Combined, those findings provide a plausible argument for the deleterious effects of hyperglycemia on articular cartilage.

An in vivo, longitudinal cohort study investigated the relationship between fasting serum glucose levels and knee structural changes in 179 adults with no knee symptoms or diagnosis of T2DM. Knee cartilage volume and presence of bone marrow lesions were assessed by MRI. Results demonstrated that tibial cartilage volume loss and incidence of bone marrow lesions were positively associated with higher levels of fasting serum glucose levels in women, but not in men.[58] The authors hypothesized that these gender differences might be owing to greater cartilage loss in women as a result of decreased levels of estrogen (a hormone that has a protective effect on cartilage) after menopause.[58]

Hyperglycemia is also known to favor the production of advanced glycation endproducts (AGEs) and their accumulation in articular cartilage, which contribute to a toxic environment that might facilitate OA pathogenesis.[59] AGE accumulation has been reported with aging, and in vitro studies demonstrated that it contributes to cartilage stiffness[60,61] and degradation.[62] High intracellular glucose concentrations in diabetes promotes formation of AGE; AGE compounds then interact with receptor of AGE to give rise to a cascade of events that promote release of proinflammatory factors such as tumor necrosis factor-α, and activate transcription factors such as nuclear factor-kB, which cause inflammation and oxidative stress intracellularly and might promote cartilage degradation.[59] AGEs may also contribute to the progression of OA through diabetic peripheral neuropathy; excess accumulation of AGEs may compromise proprioceptive and nociceptive receptors in joint structures.[63] Impaired joint proprioception has been reported in OA and postulated to be a result of dysfunctional articular mechanoreceptors and reduced muscle spindle sensitivity in weak and atrophied muscles around the joints.[64] Thus, impaired sensation in OA and diabetic neuropathy may conceal the perception of pain and further perpetuate joint damage by allowing constant harmful mechanical workloads.

It is clear that aging, obesity, and T2DM interact to affect OA (**Fig. 1**). Shared components of aging, obesity, and T2DM, such as low-grade inflammation, oxidative stress, and dysregulation of cell function, all lead to cell toxicity and consequent OA-related cartilage and bone abnormalities. Hyperglycemia also seems to have a direct effect on cartilage health. Although both lipid metabolism and vascularity play a role on joint health, the exact contribution of hypertension and dyslipidemia needs further validation.

Future Research on the Links Between Osteoarthritis and Type 2 Diabetes Mellitus

The metabolic processes linking OA and T2DM are not completely understood. We have identified several gaps in knowledge that should be addressed by future research. For example, large cross-sectional studies and longitudinal data should be used to clarify the associations between OA and T2DM prevalence and progression. These studies should apply rigorous methods to tease out the contributions of age, gender, and obesity. It is important to assess how different combinations of risk factors such as age and obesity interact with hyperglycemia to affect OA disease development, pain, and disability of patients. Moreover, although it is likely that the disruption of glucose metabolism promotes the development of OA, it could also be possible that in someone with OA, deregulated glucose metabolism just enhances the progression of OA, an issue that needs clarification. Studies should also discriminate the effects of T2DM on weight-bearing versus non–weight-bearing joints, which has not been done. Such discrimination is needed to tease out the direct contributions of hyperglycemia versus complications from T2DM, such as diabetic neuropathy, on the development and progression of OA. Last, further research is needed to clarify if and how dyslipidemia and hypertension contribute to the development of OA.

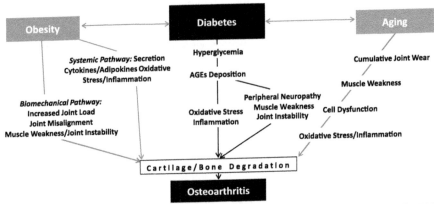

Fig. 1. Common risk factors of osteoarthritis (OA) and type 2 diabetes mellitus (T2DM). Obesity and age are well-established shared risk factors for OA and T2DM. Obesity affects OA through biomechanical and systemic pathways. Age affects OA by factors such as cumulative joint load, muscle weakness, cell dysfunction (eg, chondrocyte, mitochondria), and chronic inflammation. T2DM seems to have a direct impact on OA as hyperglycemia promotes deposition of advanced glycation end-products (AGEs) and affects cartilage health. Hyperglycemia also contributes to peripheral neuropathy, which can contribute to muscle weakness, joint instability, and consequent OA of weight-bearing joints.

Future investigations are equally needed to investigate the effects of altered glucose metabolism and AGE accumulation on cartilage health in patients with both OA and T2DM versus those with OA alone. Although studies have implicated glucose and AGE accumulation with greater severity of OA, they have not included subjects with T2DM.[65,66] Studies are necessary to confirm whether articular cartilage degradation in persons with T2DM is increased or accelerated compared with those without T2DM, which, if confirmed, could have pertinent implications for the management of these patients.

MANAGEMENT OF OLDER INDIVIDUALS WITH OSTEOARTHRITIS AND TYPE 2 DIABETES MELLITUS: A PHYSICAL ACTIVITY PERSPECTIVE

Approximately one half of all adults with diabetes have arthritis and more than one quarter of these individuals report limitation in usual activities owing to joint symptoms.[3] The functional limitations observed in older individuals with both OA and T2DM are multifactorial and involve age and obesity-related factors such as pain, muscle dysfunction (weakness, atrophy, and low quality of muscle), joint misalignment, deconditioning, poor balance and mobility, and inactivity. These limitations are exacerbated by the symptoms and complications of OA and T2DM, leading to complex interactions that further limit functional ability and compromise overall health.

A number of impairments associated with aging, OA, and T2DM develop over many years as a consequence of sedentary lifestyle and poor eating habits. Physical inactivity is a contributor to these impairments and serves as a trigger for the vicious cycle of further impairments and additional physical inactivity. Although inactivity is the trigger, physical activity is a potent intervention to break the vicious cycle. Physical activity is likely the only intervention capable of positively affecting all of the modifiable impairments listed, including the underlying pathophysiology of all of the physical impairments and symptoms. To that end, the continuation of this review focuses specifically on the management of older patients with OA who have T2DM, emphasizing the physical activity component.

Physical activity is the first-line intervention to decrease pain and functional limitations in OA. Clinical practice guidelines from the American College of Rheumatology, the American Academy of Orthopedic Surgeons, and the Osteoarthritis Research Society International have all strongly recommended that patients with symptomatic OA of the lower extremities should participate in physical activity programs that include aerobic and resistance exercises.[67–69] Regular physical activity is also one of the main treatment pillars in the management of T2DM and has been recommended by the American Diabetes Association and the American College of Sports Medicine.[70] In aging, physical activity has been recommended by the American Geriatrics Society/British Geriatrics Society and the US Department of Health and Human Services to prevent function decline.[71–73] Thus, there is solid support for the benefits of physical activity in aging, T2DM, and OA. Additionally, physical activity affects metabolism by improving glucose tolerance,[70,74–76] promoting healthy body weight, and decreasing inflammation.[77–80] Physical activity also ameliorates physical impairments, such as muscle weakness and atrophy,[81,82] joint stiffness and pain,[67–69] and poor balance and mobility.[71,73,83] Other benefits include decreased falls,[71–73] improvements in cardiovascular health,[84] improvements in mood and quality of life, and decreased mortality.[71] **Fig. 2** depicts a model for the effectiveness of physical activity on metabolic and physical impairments related to aging, OA, and T2DM.

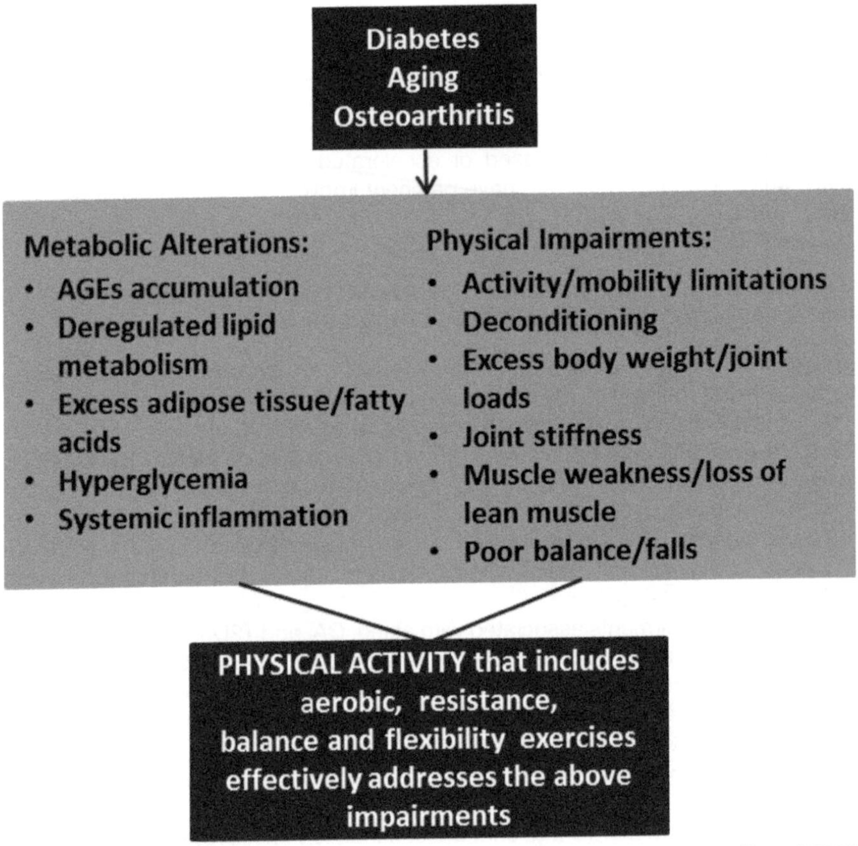

Fig. 2. Physical and metabolic impairments resultant of type 2 diabetes mellitus (T2DM), aging, and osteoarthritis (OA) that can benefit from physical activity. T2DM, aging, and OA are associated with several physical impairments and metabolic alterations that can be addressed by physical activity. Physical impairments common in this population include excess body weight and consequent increased adiposity and joint loads; poor balance and increased fall risk; muscle dysfunction such as muscle weakness, muscle atrophy, and decreased lean muscle mass; and pain and joint stiffness. All of these impairments limit daily activities and mobility. Metabolic alterations include hyperglycemia, excess adipose tissue with deregulated lipid metabolism, accumulation of advanced glycation end products (AGEs), and systemic inflammation.

Physical Activity Prescription in Older Adults with Osteoarthritis and Type 2 Diabetes Mellitus

The recommended modalities, dose, intensity, and benefits of exercise in aging, OA, and T2DM are presented in **Table 2**. These recommendations have been compiled based on clinical guidelines for the management of these patients and align with the national recommendations for physical activity.[67–71,73] It is recommended to participate in at least 150 minutes a week of aerobic activities and 2 days a week of resistive exercises. Specific to aging and OA, regular flexibility and balance exercises should also be performed.[72,83,85]

Table 2
Exercises indicated for older adults with diabetes and osteoarthritis (OA)

Modality/Examples	Dose	Intensity Level	Benefits
Aerobic exercise			
Continuous movements of large muscle groups like walking, biking, swimming, gardening, and ballroom dancing.	4–7 d per week, or every other day. Ideally, around 30 min every day. Do not go more than 2 consecutive days without exercise.	For individuals with OA of weight-bearing joints use moderate intensity. It produces noticeable increases in heart and breathing rates while person is able to engage in a conversation. For individuals without OA of weight-bearing joints, use moderate to vigorous intensity (consider overall health status).	Improves cardiovascular health, maintains body weight, improves glucose and lipid metabolism, and improves physical function.
Resistive exercise			
Activities of brief duration with weights or elastic therapy bands such as calisthenics and weight training.	2–3 d per week on nonconsecutive days. Exercise the major muscle groups of the lower extremities and trunk. Progress from 1–3 sets of 8–10 repetitions at a weight that cannot be lifted more than 8–10 times.	Moderate to high intensity resistance should allow 10–15 repetitions of each exercise, representing a perceived effort from moderate to somewhat hard.	Strengthens muscles, increases lean muscle mass, decreases fat mass, improves glucose metabolism and physical function.
Flexibility exercise			
Exercise takes the joints to their full range of pain-free motion- stretching, range of motion.	2 d per week for 10 min each day. Hold each stretch for approximately 30 s.	Light; these exercises demand low physical effort.	Maintains or increases flexibility and ameliorates joint stiffness.
Balance exercise			
Should challenge the body's dynamic stability; exercises are performed as modification of gait, such as advancing gait with changes in surfaces, rhythm, distance, load, attention, and postural transition (start, stop)- Yoga, Tai Chi, dance.	2 d per week for 15–30 min.	Light; these exercises demand low physical effort. Balance exercises require more complex control of movement and elicit postural reactions of ankle and hip joints, along with step strategies.	Improves balance and mobility, reduces fall risk and disability.

Data from Refs.[67–73]

The optimal exercise volume may need to be individually tailored to maximize benefit and safety, and minimize barriers. For example, to achieve weight loss in obesity, exercise volume ought to be larger than to achieve glycemic control and cardiovascular health. In obesity, current guidelines recommend from 250 to 300 minutes per week of aerobic exercise for weight loss and maintenance.[86] In sarcopenia, if the aim is to promote muscle hypertrophy, the intensity level of resistive training should be kept toward the high rather than the moderate range. Conversely, for individuals with severe disability the recommended volume of exercises may not be feasible and lower volume may be indicated. Although the benefits of lower volume are less compared with higher volume, emerging evidence demonstrates that low volume of exercise still promotes substantial health benefits.[87]

Although the national guidelines recommend aerobic exercises of moderate and vigorous intensities, **Table 2** differentiates the intensity of exercise according with OA weight-bearing status. In those with OA of weight-bearing joints, vigorous intensity aerobics are discouraged because they generally involve high-impact activities that could be deleterious to the joints. Moreover, many older adults with T2DM may not have sufficient aerobic capacity to undertake vigorous activities. It has also been shown that the cardiorespiratory benefits are comparable with aerobic exercises at moderate and vigorous intensities.[88–90]

When considering the type of aerobic exercise, walking has been the most widely used modality in this population. However, it is likely that walking is not as effective in obese patients with weight-bearing joint OA. In a recent literature review, we observed limited evidence for the effectiveness of walking programs on pain and physical function in patients with both obesity and OA, whereas prior studies on leaner individuals have reported beneficial effects.[91] The increased joint load combined with the increased inflammation characteristic of obesity may preclude the effectiveness of walking programs. Therefore, alternative modes such as cycling, arm ergometers, underwater walking, or water aerobics may be better choices.

Special considerations ought to be given for resistive exercises in individuals with joint pain. Resistive exercise should be performed at pain-free ranges and maximum resistance should be avoided. For example, if exercise for the knee extensor muscles cause pain at mid range (eg, 60° to 40° of knee flexion), it is recommended to try to exercise at an alternative range of motion (eg, 30° to 0°). It is also recommended that a qualified exercise trainer provide initial supervision and periodic assessment to maximize benefits and minimize injury risk of resistive exercise.[92]

Although the recommendations to exercise in **Table 2** are generic to all older adults with both OA and T2DM, some patients may be unable to follow these recommendations owing to specific impairments. For example, a patient with knee OA may present with moderate joint pain, poor balance, and weak thigh muscles; these impairments may hinder the ability to reach the recommendations. In patients like this one, alternative provisions are needed to ameliorate the physical impairment before considering more generic recommendations. It may be necessary to refer the patient to physical therapy to learn resistive exercises that target the weak muscles using pain-free ranges. Rehabilitation may also be needed to improve balance to allow the patient to safely perform exercise independently. Acquiring these new skills in rehabilitation will help the patient to engage in physical activity programs and achieve the more generic recommendations. Thus, patients who have functional limitations may need sporadic rehabilitation to resolve specific physical impairments or to adapt the exercise program to the existing physical impairments.

Special Considerations for Exercise in Older Adults with Osteoarthritis and Type 2 Diabetes Mellitus

The combination of aging, OA, and T2DM poses challenges that require particular precautions to exercise. For example, it is known that coronary artery disease is prevalent in this population and unstable disease should be brought to urgent medical attention before any exercise is instituted. Space limitations preclude us from discussing general precautions to exercise owing to other related chronic diseases. For a complete review on the relative and absolute contraindications to exercise in the general population the reader is referred elsewhere.[93,94]

Although challenges to exercise exist, the benefits of physical activity outweigh the risks. Inactivity leads to further complications and functional limitations. In general, it is safe to initiate exercise at light and moderate intensities (up to brisk walking) in this population without prior stress testing. However, it is recommended that those who are previously sedentary, have a moderate to high risk of cardiovascular disease, and want to undertake more vigorous program of physical activity should be considered for stress testing before initiating an exercise program.[95] Additionally, symptoms of exercise intolerance, such as breathlessness, muscle pain, and weakness during exercise, along with headache, nausea, dizziness, or extreme fatigue after exercise warrant specialized medical assessment. **Table 3** describes contraindications to exercise exclusively from the OA and T2DM standpoints. Whereas in OA joint pain and other signs of joint inflammation are the main criteria precluding exercise performance, in T2DM, glycemic control mainly dictates the contraindications to exercise. Contraindications related to aging are not depicted in **Table 3** because age itself is an indication for exercise rather than a contraindication. However, aging accentuates several impairments common in OA and T2DM, such as muscle weakness and poor balance and mobility; therefore, these age-related impairments should be considered to improve safety of exercise. In addition to contraindications, special considerations for exercise are also in order in this population to improve safety and comfort of exercise and those are described in **Box 1**.

Weight Loss

The focus of this segment of the review is on physical activity intervention. However, a brief discussion of weight loss in this population is warranted. Although strong evidence supports losing weight in obese individuals with OA[67,69] and in those with T2DM[92]; in older adults (older than 70 years), weight loss seems to accelerate sarcopenia.[96] Thus, we believe that for older adults with OA and T2DM, it is safe to recommend that weight loss be always accompanied by exercise to prevent loss of muscle mass. In support of this recommendation, it has been well established that the largest benefits for joint pain, metabolic impairments, and physical function have been observed in persons who exercise and lose weight.[97–100]

Exercise Adherence

Benefits from exercise are best accrued by regular physical activity participation and are likely reversible if discontinued; therefore, improving adherence to exercise is key for promoting long-term benefits. Thus, the goal is to permanently increase physical activity level. Yet, long-term maintenance of physical activity programs is a challenge, especially given the combination of chronic diseases. The presence of multiple chronic diseases or poorer mobility in individuals with OA was shown to contribute to low exercise adherence.[101]

Table 3
Contraindications to exercise in osteoarthritis and diabetes

Contraindication Type	Contraindication	Explanation
Osteoarthritis		
Relative	Mild to moderate joint pain	Most people can safely work through mild joint pain. If pain is worse 2 h after exercise, stop exercise for 1–2 d and
		Decrease amount of exercise next time
		Exercise different joints (eg, if knees hurt during walking, skip lower body training and work on upper body instead)
Absolute	Moderate to severe joint pain	Continued pressure on inflamed joints can cause further damage; switch to a workout that puts less pressure on joints (eg, swimming)
		Extreme joint pain requires further medical examination
Diabetes[73,83,92,105]		
Relative (requiring closer monitoring—based on blood glucose [BGl])	BG 70–100 mg/dL	Have a snack; 15 g of carbohydrates for every hour of moderately intense activity
	BG 100–300 mg/dL	Proceed with exercise program
	BG >300 mg/dL	If patient feels well, is adequately hydrated, and urine and/or blood ketones are negative, proceed with light- or moderate-intensity exercise with periodic monitoring of BG
		In the absence of very severe insulin deficiency, light- or moderate-intensity exercise tends to decrease BG
		If BG rises with exercise, stop exercise
Absolute		Ingestion of alcohol 3 h before exercise
		Hypoglycemia—BG <70 mg/dL. Symptoms include shakiness, pale skin color, dizziness, behavior changes, sweating, clumsy/jerky movements, hunger, seizure, headache, tingling sensations around the mouth
		Hyperglycemia—BG >300 mg/dL with ketones and >1 of the following require emergency treatment: Shortness of breath, nausea and vomiting, breath that smells fruity, a very dry mouth

Information in this table is not intended for use by patients.
Data from Refs.[67–73]

Box 1
Special considerations for exercise in aging, osteoarthritis (OA) and type 2 diabetes mellitus (T2DM)

General Considerations

- Drink plenty fluids before, during, and after exercise.

- Extended exposure to high temperature increases susceptibility to adverse effects from heat; exercise should be performed in a cool environment.

- Delayed onset muscle soreness is common in the days after exercise (when starting or progressing exercise).

- Physician assessment is required in case of development or worsening of hypertension, angina pectoris, arrhythmia, resting tachycardia, claudication, frequent oscillations in fasting glucose levels, wounds in lower extremities, muscle weakness, joint pain, and vision disturbances.

- Use of diuretics and β-blockers: high doses of diuretics can interfere with fluid and electrolyte balance whereas β-blockers can increase risk of hypoglycemia unawareness.

- For patients who take regular joint pain medication (eg, analgesics, nonsteroidal anti-inflammatory drugs), it is recommended to time the medication accordingly to decrease discomfort during exercise.

Exercise Progression

- Progression should be gradual to improve safety and to facilitate adaptation.

- Previously sedentary individuals have to gradually build up amount of exercise, starting with as little as 5–10 minutes per day.

- From the OA standpoint, exercise should progress only if patients do not experience increased joint pain, effusion, sensations of instability, or decreased joint motion.

- To reduce the likelihood of delayed onset muscle soreness, exercise should be started at low intensity and gradually increased to the target level as tolerated.

- The exercise program should be reviewed regularly and be progressed/adjusted as appropriate.

T2DM-Specific Considerations

- Maintain good diabetes control (hemoglobin A1C generally <7%).

- Carry fast acting carbohydrate at all times and ingest it if glucose levels drop.

- Carry an ID at all times with indication of medical conditions.

- Wear proper shoes and clothes according with the type of exercise.

- Perform foot inspection often.

- Insulin injection site should be rotated away from active muscles.

- For those who take insulin or insulin secretagogues, blood glucose should be checked before, after, and several hours after exercise, at least until they know their usual glycemic responses to exercise. For those with tendency to hypoglycemia, reduce medication before exercise and/or consume extra carbohydrate before exercise

In the Presence of Nephropathy

- Systolic BP should not rise above 180 mm Hg.

- Avoid weight lifting, breath holding, or high-intensity exercise.

In the Presence of Retinopathy

- Avoid vigorous activities, head jarring activities, Valsalva maneuvers, and position with the head below the waist; non–weight-bearing exercise (biking, walking in the pool, ballroom dancing) is recommended.

- Systolic BP should not rise above 20 mm Hg of resting value.

In the Presence of Autonomic Neuropathy

- Monitor signs of blood glucose and silent ischemia (eg, dyspnea, diaphoresis, orthostatic hypotension); BP and HR response to exercise may be blunted.

In the Presence of Peripheral Neuropathy

- Pain and burning can make it difficult to bear weight; do non–weight-bearing or reduced weight-bearing exercises (eg, aquatic exercises and bicycle).
- Balance and control of movement may be impaired and contribute to falls; incorporate balance exercises along with precautions to avoid falls during exercise

In the Presence of Charcot Foot

- Use a stationary or arm bike or do chair exercises using free weights.

In the Presence of Foot Ulcer and/or Deformity

- If active foot ulcer is present, perform non–weight-bearing exercise.
- Avoid swimming, keep feet clean and dry.

Abbreviations: BP, blood pressure; HR, heart rate.
Data from Refs.[73,83,92,105]

Although adherence to exercise is a complex issue beyond the scope of this review, several strategies may be helpful to promote sustainability of exercise. Efforts must be taken to engage participants and impress upon them the importance of physical activity while initiating an intervention program. Patients should be encouraged to set physical activity goals, discuss barriers to exercise, and develop strategies to overcome those barriers. To that end, self-management programs have been shown effective to educate and engage patients, and improve exercise adherence.[67–69] Exercises should also be easily instituted and individuals should engage in activities that they enjoy. Exercising at home instead of a fitness facility, and use of simple exercise mode such as walking, have shown to improve adherence.[101] Additionally, physical activity programs need to be flexible, inexpensive, fun, and not greatly interfere with a person's daily routine. Thus, perhaps the 30 minutes per day may need to be broken up into more feasible small bouts of 10 minutes walking or cycling several times a day, because this regimen is as effective as a single longer session of equivalent length and intensity.[71] Monitoring activity through diaries and activity monitors or pedometers has also been shown to increase exercise adherence.

We also believe an important hindrance to adherence to physical activity is the biases of health care professionals not to consider that OA and T2DM in older adults can be treated by physical activity. They tend to neglect the beneficial effects of exercise on cell function and on the common physiologic components of these conditions, such as systemic inflammation, hyperglycemia, and lipid metabolism. Physical activity is a powerful intervention that should be approached as a "pill" and taken as prescribed. A great advantage of this "pill" is its negligible side effects when special considerations and precautions to exercise are followed. If health care professionals prescribe the physical activity "pill" with the enthusiasm that it deserves, it would potentially improve exercise adherence.

Future Research on Physical Activity in Older Adult with Both Osteoarthritis and Type 2 Diabetes Mellitus

Although there is strong evidence for the benefits of physical activity for older adults with T2DM or OA, the evidence for exercise in individuals with a combination of these conditions is limited. After an extensive Medline search, we were unable to find studies on the effectiveness of exercise in those diagnosed with both OA and T2DM. Thus, it is unclear if the interaction of aging, OA, and T2DM would modify the response or safety of exercise. To that end, future studies are warranted to clarify several important issues. For example, if research confirms that the cartilage and subchondral bone of patients with T2DM are more prone to damage, it will likely prompt adaptations to exercise prescription in this population. Intervention studies should investigate the (1) dose–response of exercise, particularly the safety of weight-bearing exercises, (2) effects of exercise on cartilage and subchondral bone health, (3) consequences of increased joint loads in well controlled-versus not well-controlled T2DM, (4) safety of weight loss interventions, and (5) optimal combinations of aerobic and strength exercise to improve physical function and decrease pain.

SUMMARY

Emerging evidence supports that people with T2DM are more susceptible to develop arthritis. OA and T2DM in aging are linked by age and obesity factors, such as cumulative joint loads, systemic inflammation, and abnormal lipid metabolism. Hyperglycemia may also directly impact OA. In this review, we have discussed the common links between OA and T2DM in older adults along with the metabolic and physical impairments commonly present in this population. We emphasized the role of physical activity and the only intervention capable of addressing a large number of metabolic and physical impairments in older adults with both OA and T2DM.

REFERENCES

1. Lawrence RC, Felson DT, Helmick CG, et al. Estimates of the prevalence of arthritis and other rheumatic conditions in the United States. Part II. Arthritis Rheum 2008;58(1):26–35.
2. US Centers for Disease Control and Prevention. National diabetes statistics report, 2014. Estimates of diabetes and its burden in the United States fact sheet. Available at: http://www.cdc.gov/diabetes/pubs/estimates14.htm. Accessed July 14, 2014.
3. Prevalence of doctor-diagnosed arthritis and arthritis-attributable activity limitation – United States, 2007-2009. MMWR Morb Mortal Wkly Rep 2010;59(39): 1261–5.
4. Centers for Disease Control and Prevention. 2011 national diabetes fact sheet. 2011. Available at: http://www.cdc.gov/diabetes/pubs/factsheet11.htm. Accessed February 10, 2014.
5. Schett G, Kleyer A, Perricone C, et al. Diabetes is an independent predictor for severe osteoarthritis: results from a longitudinal cohort study. Diabetes Care 2013;36(2):403–9.
6. Sturmer TB, Brenner RE, Gunther KP. Non-insulin dependent diabetes mellitus (NIDDM) and patterns of osteoarthritis. Scand J Rheumatol 2001;30:169–71.
7. Arthritis as a potential barrier to physical activity among adults with diabetes - United States, 2005 and 2007. MMWR Morb Mortal Wkly Rep 2008;57(18): 486–9.
8. Waine H, Nevinny D, Rosenthal J, et al. Association of osteoarthritis and diabetes mellitus. Tufts Folia Med 1961;7:13–9.
9. Cnop M, Igiollo-Esteve M, Hughes SJ, et al. Longevity of human islet α-and β-cells. Diabetes Obes Metab 2001;13(Suppl 1):39–46.

10. Berenbaum F. Diabetes-induced osteoarthritis: from a new paradigm to a new phenotype. Ann Rheum Dis 2011;70(8):1354–6.

11. Harman D. Aging: a theory based on free radical and radiation chemistry. J Gerontol 1956;11(3):298–300.

12. Harman D. The biologic clock: the mitochondria? J Am Geriatr Soc 1972;20(4): 145–7.

13. Trounce I, Byrne E, Marzuki S. Decline in skeletal muscle mitochondrial respiratory chain function: possible factor in ageing. Lancet 1989;1(8639): 637–9.

14. Kahn SE, Hull RL, Utzschneider KM. Mechanisms linking obesity to insulin resistance and type 2 diabetes. Nature 2006;444(7121):840–6.

15. Goldring MB. Osteoarthritis and cartilage: the role of cytokines. Curr Rheumatol Rep 2000;2(6):459–65.

16. Felson DT, Zhang Y, Hannan MT, et al. Risk factors for incident radiographic knee osteoarthritis in the elderly: the Framingham study. Arthritis Rheum 1997; 40(4):728–33.

17. Reijman M, Pols HA, Bergink AP, et al. Body mass index associated with onset and progression of osteoarthritis of the knee but not of the hip: the Rotterdam study. Ann Rheum Dis 2007;66(2):158–62.

18. Sharma L, Lou C, Cahue S, et al. The mechanism of the effect of obesity in knee osteoarthritis: the mediating role of malalignment. Arthritis Rheum 2000;43(3): 568–75.

19. Syed IY, Davis BL. Obesity and osteoarthritis of the knee: hypotheses concerning the relationship between ground reaction forces and quadriceps fatigue in long-duration walking. Med Hypotheses 2000;54(2):182–5.

20. Slemenda C, Heilman DK, Brandt KD, et al. Reduced quadriceps strength relative to body weight: a risk factor for knee osteoarthritis in women? Arthritis Rheum 1998;41(11):1951–9.

21. Sellam J, Berenbaum F. Is osteoarthritis a metabolic disease? Joint Bone Spine 2013;80(6):568–73.

22. Fernandes JC, Martel-Pelletier J, Pelletier JP. The role of cytokines in osteoarthritis pathophysiology. Biorheology 2002;39(1–2):237–46.

23. Toda Y, Toda T, Takemura S, et al. Change in body fat, but not body weight or metabolic correlates of obesity, is related to symptomatic relief of obese patients with knee osteoarthritis after a weight control program. J Rheumatol 1998; 25(11):2181–6.

24. Dumond H, Presle N, Terlain B, et al. Evidence for a key role of leptin in osteoarthritis. Arthritis Rheum 2003;48(11):3118–29.

25. Koskinen A, Vuolteenaho K, Nieminen R, et al. Leptin enhances MMP-1, MMP-3 and MMP-13 production in human osteoarthritic cartilage and correlates with MMP-1 and MMP-3 in synovial fluid from OA patients. Clin Exp Rheumatol 2011;29(1):57–64.

26. Filkova M, Liskova M, Hulejova H, et al. Increased serum adiponectin levels in female patients with erosive compared with non-erosive osteoarthritis. Ann Rheum Dis 2009;68(2):295–6.

27. Yusuf E, Ioan-Facsinay A, Bijsterbosch J, et al. Association between leptin, adiponectin and resistin and long-term progression of hand osteoarthritis. Ann Rheum Dis 2011;70(7):1282–4.

28. Conde J, Scotece M, Gomez R, et al. Adipokines and osteoarthritis: novel molecules involved in the pathogenesis and progression of disease. Arthritis 2011;2011:203901.

29. National High Blood Pressure Education Program Working Group. National High Blood Pressure Education Program Working Group report on hypertension in diabetes. Hypertension 1994;23:145–58.
30. Fukui M, Tanaka M, Toda H, et al. Risk factors for development of diabetes mellitus, hypertension and dyslipidemia. Diabetes Res Clin Pract 2011;94(1):e15–8.
31. Hart DJ, Doyle DV, Spector TD. Association between metabolic factors and knee osteoarthritis in women: the Chingford study. J Rheumatol 1995;22:1118–23.
32. Velasquez MT, Katz JD. Osteoarthritis: another component of metabolic syndrome? Metab Syndr Relat Disord 2010;8(4):295–305.
33. Zhuo Q, Yang W, Chen J, et al. Metabolic syndrome meets osteoarthritis. Nat Rev Rheumatol 2012;8(12):729–37.
34. Findlay DM. Vascular pathology and osteoarthritis. Rheumatology 2007;46(12): 1763–8.
35. Puenpatom RA, Victor TW. Increased prevalence of metabolic syndrome in individuals with osteoarthritis: an analysis of NHANES III data. Postgrad Med 2009; 121(6):9–20.
36. Engstrom G, Gerhardsson de Verdier M, Rollof J, et al. C-reactive protein, metabolic syndrome and incidence of severe hip and knee osteoarthritis. A population-based cohort study. Osteoarthr Cartil 2009;17(2):168–73.
37. Marks R, Allegrante JP. Comorbid disease profiles of adults with end-stage hip osteoarthritis. Med Sci Monit 2002;8(4):CR305–9.
38. Conaghan PG, Vanharanta H, Dieppe PA. Is progressive osteoarthritis an atheromatous vascular disease? Ann Rheum Dis 2005;64(11):1539–41.
39. Lippiello L, Walsh T, Fienhold M. The association of lipid abnormalities with tissue pathology in human osteoarthritic articular cartilage. Metabolism 1991; 40(6):571–6.
40. Gkretsi V, Simopoulou T, Tsezou A. Lipid metabolism and osteoarthritis: lessons from atherosclerosis. Prog Lipid Res 2011;50(2):133–40.
41. Simopoulou T, Malizos KN, Tsezou A. Lectin-like oxidized low density lipoprotein receptor 1 (LOX-1) expression in human articular chondrocytes. Clin Exp Rheumatol 2007;25(4):605–12.
42. Wang Y, Wluka AE, Hodge AM, et al. Effect of fatty acids on bone marrow lesions and knee cartilage in healthy, middle-aged subjects without clinical knee osteoarthritis. Osteoarthr Cartil 2008;16(5):579–83.
43. Plumb MS, Aspden RM. High levels of fat and (n-6) fatty acids in cancellous bone in osteoarthritis. Lipids Health Dis 2004;3:12.
44. Felson DT, McLaughlin S, Goggins J, et al. Bone marrow edema and its relation to progression of knee osteoarthritis. Ann Intern Med 2003;139(5 Pt 1):330–6.
45. Clark BC, Manini TM. Functional consequences of sarcopenia and dynapenia in the elderly. Curr Opin Clin Nutr Metab Care 2010;13(3):271–6.
46. Hulens M, Vansant G, Claessens AL, et al. Predictors of 6-minute walk test results in lean, obese and morbidly obese women. Scand J Med Sci Sports 2003;13(2):98–105.
47. Melissas J, Kontakis G, Volakakis E, et al. The effect of surgical weight reduction on functional status in morbidly obese patients with low back pain. Obes Surg 2005;15(3):378–81.
48. Hills AP, Hennig EM, McDonald M, et al. Plantar pressure differences between obese and non-obese adults: a biomechanical analysis. Int J Obes Relat Metab Disord 2001;25(11):1674–9.
49. Barofsky I, Fontaine KR, Cheskin LJ. Pain in the obese: impact on health-related quality-of-life. Ann Behav Med 1997;19(4):408–10.

50. Frey MI, Barrett-Connor E, Sledge PA, et al. The effect of noninsulin dependent diabetes mellitus on the prevalence of clinical osteoarthritis: a population based study. J Rheumatol 1996;23(4):716–22.
51. Horn CA, Bradley JD, Brandt KD, et al. Osteophyte formation in diabetic patients with OA. Arthritis Rheum 1992;35(3):336–42.
52. Nieves-Plaza M, Castro-Santana LE, Font YM, et al. Association of hand or knee osteoarthritis with diabetes mellitus in a population of Hispanics from Puerto Rico. J Clin Rheumatol 2013;19(1):1–6.
53. Mobasheri A, Vannucci SJ, Bondy CA, et al. Glucose transport and metabolism in chondrocytes: a key to understanding chondrogenesis, skeletal development and cartilage degradation in osteoarthritis. Histol Histopathol 2002;17(4):1239–67.
54. Rosa SC, Goncalves J, Judas F, et al. Impaired glucose transporter-1 degradation and increased glucose transport and oxidative stress in response to high glucose in chondrocytes from osteoarthritic versus normal human cartilage. Arthritis Res Ther 2009;11(3):R80.
55. Yan W, Li X. Impact of diabetes and its treatments on skeletal diseases. Front Med 2013;7(1):81–90.
56. Goldring MB. Update on the biology of the chondrocyte and new approaches to treating cartilage diseases. Best Pract Res Clin Rheumatol 2006;20(5):1003–25.
57. Rosa SC, Rufino AT, Judas FM, et al. Role of glucose as a modulator of anabolic and catabolic gene expression in normal and osteoarthritic human chondrocytes. J Cell Biochem 2011;112(10):2813–24.
58. Davies-Tuck ML, Wang Y, Wluka AE, et al. Increased fasting serum glucose concentration is associated with adverse knee structural changes in adults with no knee symptoms and diabetes. Maturitas 2012;72(4):373–8.
59. Brownlee M. Biochemistry and molecular cell biology of diabetic complications. Nature 2001;414(6865):813–20.
60. Verzijl N, DeGroot J, Ben ZC, et al. Crosslinking by advanced glycation end products increases the stiffness of the collagen network in human articular cartilage: a possible mechanism through which age is a risk factor for osteoarthritis. Arthritis Rheum 2002;46(1):114–23.
61. Verzijl N, DeGroot J, Oldehinkel E, et al. Age-related accumulation of Maillard reaction products in human articular cartilage collagen. Biochem J 2000;350(Pt 2):381–7.
62. Steenvoorden MM, Huizinga TW, Verzijl N, et al. Activation of receptor for advanced glycation end products in osteoarthritis leads to increased stimulation of chondrocytes and synoviocytes. Arthritis Rheum 2006;54(1):253–63.
63. Leaverton PE, Peregoy J, Fahlman L, et al. Does diabetes hide osteoarthritis pain? Med Hypotheses 2012;78(4):471–4.
64. Knoop J, Steultjens MP, Leeden M, et al. Proprioception in knee osteoarthritis: a narrative review. 2011. Osteoarthr Cartil 2011;19:381–8.
65. Nakamura H, Masuko K, Yudoh K, et al. Positron emission tomography with 18F-FDG in osteoarthritic knee. Osteoarthr Cartil 2007;15(6):673–81.
66. Hong YH, Kong EJ. (18F)Fluoro-deoxy-D-glucose uptake of knee joints in the aspect of age- related osteoarthritis: a case-control study. BMC Musculoskelet Disord 2013;14:141.
67. Jevsevar DS. Treatment of osteoarthritis of the knee: evidence-based guideline, 2nd edition. J Am Acad Orthop Surg 2013;21(9):571–6.
68. Zhang W, Moskowitz RW, Nuki G, et al. OARSI recommendations for the management of hip and knee osteoarthritis, Part II: OARSI evidence-based, expert consensus guidelines. Osteoarthr Cartil 2008;16(2):137–62.

69. Hochberg MC, Altman RD, April KT, et al. American College of Rheumatology 2012 recommendations for the use of nonpharmacologic and pharmacologic therapies in osteoarthritis of the hand, hip, and knee. Arthritis Care Res 2012; 64(4):465–74.

70. Colberg SR, Albright AL, Blissmer BJ, et al. Exercise and type 2 diabetes: American College of Sports Medicine and the American Diabetes Association: joint position statement. Exercise and type 2 diabetes. Med Sci Sports Exerc 2010;42(12):2282–303.

71. US Department of Health and Human Services. 2008 Physical activity guidelines for Americans. Available at: http://www.health.gov/paguidelines/. Accessed February 11, 2014.

72. Agency for Healthcare Research and Quality. Physical activity and older Americans: benefits and strategies. Available at: http://www.innovations.ahrq.gov/content.aspx?id=991. Accessed February 11, 2014.

73. Panel on Prevention of Falls in Older Persons, American Geriatrics Society, and British Geriatrics Society. Summary of the updated American Geriatrics Society/British Geriatrics Society clinical practice guideline for prevention of falls in older persons. J Am Geriatr Soc 2011;59(1):148–57.

74. Coker RH, Williams RH, Yeo SE, et al. The impact of exercise training compared to caloric restriction on hepatic and peripheral insulin resistance in obesity. J Clin Endocrinol Metab 2009;94(11):4258–66.

75. Haus JM, Solomon TP, Marchetti CM, et al. Free fatty acid-induced hepatic insulin resistance is attenuated following lifestyle intervention in obese individuals with impaired glucose tolerance. J Clin Endocrinol Metab 2010;95(1): 323–7.

76. Solomon TP, Haus JM, Marchetti CM, et al. Effects of exercise training and diet on lipid kinetics during free fatty acid-induced insulin resistance in older obese humans with impaired glucose tolerance. Am J Physiol Endocrinol Metab 2009; 297(2):E552–9.

77. Balducci S, Zanuso S, Nicolucci A, et al. Anti-inflammatory effect of exercise training in subjects with type 2 diabetes and the metabolic syndrome is dependent on exercise modalities and independent of weight loss. Nutr Metab Cardiovasc Dis 2010;20(8):608–17.

78. Donges CE, Duffield R, Drinkwater EJ. Effects of resistance or aerobic exercise training on interleukin-6, C-reactive protein, and body composition. Med Sci Sports Exerc 2010;42(2):304–13.

79. Smart NA, Larsen AI, Le Maitre JP, et al. Effect of exercise training on interleukin-6, tumour necrosis factor alpha and functional capacity in heart failure. Cardiol Res Pract 2011;2011:532620.

80. Conraads VM, Beckers P, Bosmans J, et al. Combined endurance/resistance training reduces plasma TNF-alpha receptor levels in patients with chronic heart failure and coronary artery disease. Eur Heart J 2002;23(23):1854–60.

81. Hansen D, Dendale P, van Loon LJ, et al. The impact of training modalities on the clinical benefits of exercise intervention in patients with cardiovascular disease risk or type 2 diabetes mellitus. Sports Med 2010;40(11):921–40.

82. Weinheimer EM, Sands LP, Campbell WW. A systematic review of the separate and combined effects of energy restriction and exercise on fat-free mass in middle-aged and older adults: implications for sarcopenic obesity. Nutr Rev 2010;68(7):375–88.

83. McDermott AY, Mernitz H. Exercise and older patients: prescribing guidelines. Am Fam Physician 2006;74(3):437–44.

84. Williams MA, Haskell WL, Ades PA, et al. Resistance exercise in individuals with and without cardiovascular disease: 2007 update: a scientific statement from the American Heart Association Council on Clinical Cardiology and Council on Nutrition, Physical Activity, and Metabolism. Circulation 2007;116(5):572–84.

85. Elsawy B, Higgins KE. Physical activity guidelines for older adults. Am Fam Physician 2010;81(1):55–9.

86. Donnelly JE, Blair SN, Jakicic JM, et al. American College of Sports Medicine Position Stand. Appropriate physical activity intervention strategies for weight loss and prevention of weight regain for adults. Med Sci Sports Exerc 2009; 41(2):459–71.

87. Sattelmair J, Pertman J, Ding EL, et al. Dose response between physical activity and risk of coronary heart disease: a meta-analysis. Circulation 2011;124(7): 789–95.

88. Kraus WE, Slentz CA. Exercise training, lipid regulation, and insulin action: a tangled web of cause and effect. Obesity (Silver Spring) 2009;17(Suppl 3): S21–6.

89. Hansen TM, Hansen G, Langgaard AM, et al. Longterm physical training in rheumatoid arthritis. A randomized trial with different training programs and blinded observers. Scand J Rheumatol 1993;22(3):107–12.

90. Slentz CA, Houmard JA, Kraus WE. Exercise, abdominal obesity, skeletal muscle, and metabolic risk: evidence for a dose response. Obesity 2009;17(Suppl 3):S27–33.

91. Khoja SS, Susko AM, Josbeno DA, et al. Comparing physical activity programs for managing osteoarthritis in overweight or obese patients. J Comp Eff Res 2014;3(3):283–99.

92. American Diabetes Association. Standards of medical care in diabetes–2007. Diabetes Care 2007;30(Suppl 1):S4–41.

93. Balady GJ, Arena R, Sietsema K, et al. Clinician's guide to cardiopulmonary exercise testing in adults: a scientific statement from the American Heart Association. Circulation 2010;122(2):191–225.

94. Thompson WR, Gordan NF, Prescatello LS. ACSM's guidelines for exercise testing and prescription. Baltimore (MD): Lippincott Williams and Wilkins; 2010.

95. Hansen D, Peeters S, Zwaenepoel B, et al. Exercise assessment and prescription in patients with type 2 diabetes in the private and home care setting: clinical recommendations from AXXON (Belgian Physical Therapy Association). Phys Ther 2013;93(5):597–610.

96. Newman AB, Lee JS, Visser M, et al. Weight change and the conservation of lean mass in old age: the health, aging and body composition study. Am J Clin Nutr 2005;82(4):872–8 [quiz: 915–6].

97. Messier SP, Loeser RF, Miller GD, et al. Exercise and dietary weight loss in overweight and obese older adults with knee osteoarthritis: the arthritis, diet, and activity promotion trial. Arthritis Rheum 2004;50(5):1501–10.

98. Messier SP, Mihalko SL, Legault C, et al. Effects of intensive diet and exercise on knee joint loads, inflammation, and clinical outcomes among overweight and obese adults with knee osteoarthritis: the IDEA randomized clinical trial. JAMA 2013;310(12):1263–73.

99. Miller GD, Nicklas BJ, Davis C, et al. Intensive weight loss program improves physical function in older obese adults with knee osteoarthritis. Obesity (Silver Spring) 2006;14(7):1219–30.

100. Chomentowski P, Dube JJ, Amati F, et al. Moderate exercise attenuates the loss of skeletal muscle mass that occurs with intentional caloric restriction-induced

weight loss in older, overweight to obese adults. J Gerontol A Biol Sci Med Sci 2009;64(5):575–80.

101. van Gool CH, Penninx BW, Kempen GI, et al. Determinants of high and low attendance to diet and exercise interventions among overweight and obese older adults. Results from the arthritis, diet, and activity promotion trial. Contemp Clin Trials 2006;27(3):227–37.

102. Herrero-Beaumont G, Roman-Blas JA, Castaneda S, et al. Primary osteoarthritis no longer primary: three subsets with distinct etiological, clinical, and therapeutic characteristics. Semin Arthritis Rheum 2009;39(2):71–80.

103. Mayo Clinic. Risk factors for diabetes. 2013. Available at: http://www.mayoclinic. org/diseases- conditions/diabetes/basics/risk-factors/con-20033091. Accessed January 2, 2014.

104. Centers for Disease Control and Prevention. Osteoarthritis risk factors. 2014. Available at: http://www.cdc.gov/arthritis/basics/risk-factors.htm. Accessed January 2, 2014.

105. Sigal RJ, Kenny GP, Wasserman DH, et al. Physical activity/exercise and type 2 diabetes: a consensus statement from the American Diabetes Association. Diabetes Care 2006;29(6):1433–8.

Falls Risk in Older Adults with Type 2 Diabetes

Aaron I. Vinik, MD, PhD[a,*], Etta J. Vinik, MA(Ed)[a], Sheri R. Colberg, PhD[b], Steven Morrison, PhD[c]

KEYWORDS

- Falls • Type 2 diabetes • Older adults • Risk

KEY POINTS

- Falls are a major health issue for older adults, leading to adverse events and even death.
- Older persons with type 2 diabetes are at an increased risk of falling compared with healthy adults of a similar age.
- More than 400 factors are associated with falls risk, making identification and targeting of key factors to prevent falls problematic.
- In addition to age- and diabetes-related factors like diminished strength and sensation (caused by peripheral neuropathy), declines in cognitive function and use of multiple prescription medications (polypharmacy) are leading reasons for increased risk of falling.
- Designing specific interventions to target physiologic functions will produce the greatest benefit for reducing falls in older persons with diabetes.

INTRODUCTION

The older adult is often faced with a myriad of health-related issues, and problems with falling is one major concern for persons older than 65 years. The outcomes of a fall are many, extending from short-term health problems (eg, lacerations, fractures, and traumatic brain injury) to long-term consequences (eg, declines in muscle strength, physical activity, increased fatigue, and heightened fear of falling).[1] In 2010, the Centers for Disease Control reported that 2.3 million older adults were treated in emergency departments for nonfatal fall-related injuries. Furthermore, falls and any fall-related consequences have been reported to be the leading cause of injury-related death and hospitalization in adults older than 65 years; a staggering one-third of persons this age who fall are likely to suffer one of these adverse events within a given year. Given the range of health issues that can arise following a fall, prevention should be the first course of action.

[a] Strelitz Diabetes Center, Eastern Virginia Medical School, 855 W Brambleton Avenue, Norfolk, VA 23510, USA; [b] Human Movement Sciences Department, Old Dominion University, 5115 Hampton Boulevard, Norfolk, VA 23529, USA; [c] School of Physical Therapy and Athletic Training, Old Dominion University, 5115 Hampton Boulevard, Norfolk, VA 23529, USA
* Corresponding author.
E-mail address: vinikai@evms.edu

Clin Geriatr Med 31 (2015) 89–99
http://dx.doi.org/10.1016/j.cger.2014.09.002   geriatric.theclinics.com

The key to preventing such an adverse event is the identification of persons at risk and implementing the appropriate intervention. This approach requires recognizing those variables or elements that can lead to an increased risk of falling. However, despite our understanding of the seriousness of falls and the high cost of medical care, identifying a few critical factors that are strongly predictive of falls in high-risk populations is lacking, partly because more than 400 are linked with falls in adult populations.[2] Even something as simple as an individual's perception of threat around them when they move (often referred to as a *fear of falling*) can be a significant health issue. Nearly 13 million (36%) older American adults (greater than 65 years of age) have been found to be moderately or very afraid of falling, illustrating that developing a fear of suffering an adverse event is strongly linked with actual falls.[3]

THE CAUSES OF FALLS

Identification of a manageable number of key risk factors for falls is not a trivial or simple undertaking. Some variables identified as significant provide little direct benefit to the older person who suffers a fall and/or the clinician because they cannot be easy implemented into a meaningful practice. For example, the most powerful predictor of a fall is a previous fall; the likelihood of a person falling in the future increases dramatically if he or she has suffered such an event in the past.[2,4] However, this variable does not identify the person who has not fallen but may be at an increased risk. This measure also provides little guidance or detail about the causes of prior falls. If the ultimate aim is to intervene before such an event occurs, then the use of previous falls history is of limited use as it provides no direction regarding identification of risk factors for falls. Ideally, the best strategy is to identify those persons at risk before a fall and intervene in a meaningful fashion to reduce their risk of falling.

RISK OF FALLING IS INCREASED FOR OLDER ADULTS WITH TYPE 2 DIABETES

- Persons with type 2 diabetes are at increased risk of falling compared with healthy adults of a similar age. A combination of age (>65 years) and diabetes increases the risk of falling 17-fold.[5,6]
- In addition to age- and diabetes-related factors like diminished sensation (caused by neuropathy), declines in cognitive function, and use of multiple prescription medications (polypharmacy) (see the article by Peron and colleagues elsewhere in this issue that also highlights the problem and its consequences for older persons with type 2 Diabetes Mellitus) are leading reasons for increased risk.[2,7,8]

The likelihood of suffering a fall increases dramatically with increasing age and/or the emergence of type 2 diabetes, with the risk being increased significantly by the presence of diabetes alone.[2,9–15] Older persons with diabetes must contend with both age-related declines in balance control, muscle strength (sarcopenia), walking ability, and proprioception[7,8,16–18] *and* health-related issues associated with diabetes.[19–22] Indeed, the additional range of potential risk factors in anyone with diabetes is quite extensive, covering nerve-related damage or impairment (neuropathy), visual deficits, loss of coordination, cognitive impairment, autonomic dysfunction with orthostatic hypotension, tachycardia, bradycardia, pain, poor lower body function, high body mass index, cardiovascular syncope, vestibular dysfunction, frontal cortex dysfunction, and use of various medications, all of which may interact and can have an additive effect.[2,17,18,23,24] Thus, the older person with diabetes typically has a significantly greater risk of suffering a fall when compared with a healthy adult of similar age.[5,20,22] **Fig. 1** illustrates the pattern of increase in the falls risk as a function of increasing age and the development of type 2 diabetes.

NEUROPATHY IS STRONGLY LINKED TO FALLING

Declines in sensory function arising from neuropathy are a major contributing factor to the overall increase in the falls risk factor for persons with diabetes.[19,23,25–27] In fact, diabetic neuropathies (DN) can affect up to 50% of people with type 2 diabetes, contributing to increased mortality and loss of quality of life.[28] These neuropathies are a heterogeneous set of conditions that involve different aspects of the somatic and autonomic nervous systems, including small and large fiber peripheral and auto-nomic nerves. Some of the principal factors contributing to DN include chronic hyper-glycemia, microvascular insufficiency, oxidative stress, greater height, and advancing age.[28]

Arguably the most common form of neuropathy is distal, symmetric, diabetic poly-neuropathy (DPN), which affects peripheral sensory and motor function and can be found in around 40% to 100% of diabetic individuals.[28] Consequences of DPN extend to decrements in balance and altered walking function,[29–32] which are obvious medi-ators for an increased falls risk.[17,19,27,33,34] The ability to optimally control one's bal-ance is essential for mobility, avoidance of disability, and preservation of independence in older people.[35] The complexity of the balance system makes local-ization of the problem difficult because the abnormality may occur in one or more of

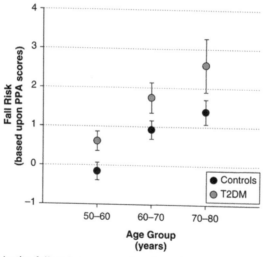

Fig. 1. Differences in the falls risk score as a function of age (50–60 years, 60–70 years, and 70–80 years) and disease status (healthy older adults [controls] and older adults with type 2 diabetes). The falls risk of each person was assessed using the Physiologic Profile Assessment (PPA). The PPA consists of a battery of physiologic measures covering tests of vision (edge contrast sensitivity, high/low contrast visual acuity, depth perception), sensation (ankle touch sensitivity, leg proprioception), reaction time (from the hand and foot), leg strength (knee flexion and extension, ankle dorsi-flexion), postural sway, and balance coordination. Values from each test are combined to provide an overall risk score, which range from −2 (very low risk) to +4 (marked risk).[4,18] For each age group, falls risk values are compared against age-matched normative values. Mean values are shown for each group. Error bars represent one standard error of the mean. TD2M, type 2 diabetes mellitus.

the sensory sites (vision, vestibular, somatosensory) or in the motor system. A thorough evaluation of the sensory-motor systems affecting balance is required to arrive at a diagnosis and to create a platform to provide a menu for treatment and management choices.

Because neuropathy progression follows a distal-to-proximal gradient, the effects of DPN on strength and balance are most evident at the ankles and feet, sites of the distal endings of large, myelinated motor and sensory fibers. The loss of nerve function can have dramatic implications for both standing and walking tasks.[35] For example, diabetic persons with sensory deficits in the feet can exhibit increased postural motion and slower gait speed[29–32] with increased stride time variability.[26,30,36–41] Their impact is further magnified when the task is made more difficult, as when walking or standing on irregular surfaces.[19,42,43]

In addition, there is slowing of the reaction time, loss of the ability to prevent progression to a fall after its initiation, and dorsiflexion weakness,[44] which increase the susceptibility to tripping on loose rugs, carpets, and minor variations in step height (eg, the first step or last step on a flight of stairs). Although older adults with diabetes are a heterogeneous group, ranging from fit and healthy to frail with many comorbidities and functional disabilities, poorly controlled diabetes with polyuria escalates the falls risk simply because of the number of visits to and urgency to use the bathroom.[20,22–24]

CHANGES IN COGNITIVE FUNCTION ARE LINKED TO FALLS

The risk factors for falling are not simply confined to those variables associated with sensory-motor function. Cognitive decline, particularly related to executive functioning, is a contributing factor to instability. A recent report from the American Geriatrics Society stressed the significance of any decline in cognitive function for falling, with approximately 60% of older persons with cognitive impairment reporting a fall each year.[45] Falls in older people are associated with changes in the prefrontal cortex leading to failures of executive control.[46] Gait performance, particularly changes in stride time variability, has been associated with changes in executive function.[47]

Changes in cognitive function also extend to a person's perception of threats in the environment. If an individual perceives himself or herself to be unstable and at risk of falling, he or she may co-contract (stiffen) the leg muscles to remain stable, adjust his or her gait by walking slower, and reducing step length.[48–50] This perception of instability is referred to as *fear of falling*.[3,51–53] Those who develop a fear of falling often further self-limit their activities, leading to reduced mobility, physical fitness, and increasing the risk of falling.[54,55] Ironically, although older people recognize the benefits of activity for reducing their falls risk, many with increased fear of falling reduce their activity even without an underlying injury or medical reason for doing so.[3] Thus, fear of falling is a major confounding factor to consider when assessing the falls risk.

THE PROBLEM OF POLYPHARMACY

In addition to the general physiologic changes often seen with increasing age and disease, the high incidence of polypharmacy (ie, 4 or more medications)[56] (also see the article by Peron and colleagues elsewhere in this issue) is another major risk factor for falls,[57–59] one that needs to be addressed to lower the risk. Research has shown that a simple reduction of psychotropic medications and polypharmacy can result in a significantly reduced fall rate.[60,61] In healthy, nonfrail individuals with a greater than 5-year life expectancy, health management goals should be similar to those of the young.[62] However, in frail, elderly patients with diabetes, avoidance of hypoglycemia, hypotension, and drug interactions caused by polypharmacy are of even greater concern.[63] The accompanying review by Peron and colleagues elsewhere in this issue also highlights the problem and its consequences for older persons with type 2 diabetes mellitus.

Proper management of coexisting medical conditions is important, as it influences their ability to perform self-management. Hyperglycemia increases dehydration and impairs vision and cognition,[64] all of which contribute to functional decline and should be avoided in elderly, diabetic patients. However, side effects of diabetes treatment, most notably hypoglycemia, can result in poor outcomes, such as traumatic falls and exacerbation of comorbid conditions. Similarly, reduction of psychotropic medications and polypharmacy has been shown to also result in a reduced fall rate.[8,20,57,65,66] Depression is another cognitive factor commonly associated with falls and diabetes because of increased activity avoidance and the prescription of psychotropic medications to treat this disorder.[8,20,57,59]

Furthermore, the delicacy of electrolyte balance in older people and the use of diuretics and other drugs causing hyponatremia (serum sodium <135 mmol/L) are increasingly recognized as risk factors. Hyponatremia is associated with gait disturbances, decreased mentation, and falls. Among older patients admitted to the emergency department with asymptomatic, chronic hyponatremia, the incidence of falls was 21.3% in the hyponatremic group compared with 5.3% in controls; the former group demonstrated highly unstable gait and attention impairment that were completely reversed with correction of hyponatremia.[67] Although mild hyponatremia can result in an unsteady gait, cognitive impairment, and falls by inducing subtle neurologic changes,[68] it likely also directly contributes to development of osteoporosis and increased bone fragility by inducing increased bone resorption to mobilize sodium.[69] Given that the most common potentially causative factors in cases of hyponatremia are the use of thiazide diuretics (76%), dehydration (70%), and use of proton pump inhibitors (70%), clinicians should check for the presence of hyponatremia and treat it to prevent falls and fractures.[69]

WHAT INTERVENTIONS WORK BEST FOR REDUCING FALLS RISK?

Recent Cochrane reports cited the development and tailoring of interventions specific to the population group at risk as the issue of most significance in reducing falls.[70,71] As most falls occur during movement, identifying factors that negatively impact balance and/or walking ability is critical. Some variables directly affect the components involved in dynamic balance control (eg, muscle strength, coordination, sensory loss, blood pressure, and pain management), whereas others can affect balance indirectly by altering the postural processes underlying balance control (eg, polypharmacy, urinary incontinence, dementia, mild cognitive impairment, mild hypoglycemia and hypoglycemia autonomic failure, and depressive symptoms).

- In order to have a positive effect on the falls risk, only those measures that can be modified should be targeted in interventions.
- Various approaches in persons with diabetes can likely reduce falls, such as a reduced intensity of glycemic control, less stringent blood pressure lowering, reduction of polypharmacy, and treatment of neuropathic symptoms (including pain management).
- Physiologic variables, such as those underlying strength and balance ability, can be effectively targeted with different exercise interventions.

- The introduction of medical nutrition therapy, including possible replacement of vitamin B_{12} and vitamin D, may be beneficial.

Of the numerous falls risk factors identified, those of greater significance tend to be impaired balance and mobility related to age-related declines in physiologic functioning.[70] Consequently, most screening tools and interventions have been specifically designed to target balance, walking dysfunction, reactions, and muscle weakness because they are modifiable in older adults and most likely to be positively influence by tailored interventions. For example, exercise can lead to improvements in body composition and arthritic pain, reduced falls risk and depression, increased strength and balance, improved quality of life, and improved survival for older persons.[72–74] **Fig. 2** diagrams the link between screening assessments and potential interventions. Ideally, a person at an increased risk should be directed to an intervention designed specific to the major risk factor.

Studies of frail elderly people have shown that weight training should be included in addition to aerobic exercises.[75] Although numerous studies have shown the benefits of various balance/exercise programs in reducing the falls risk in healthy older persons,[13,71,76–78] there have been surprisingly few studies of the benefits of this form of intervention for reducing the falls risk in the diabetic population. Those studies performed have reported that targeted interventions can improve both balance and walking ability and reduce the falls risk.[17,18,79] Structured balance training can lead to general improvements in posture and/or gait function[17,18,80] as well as general gains

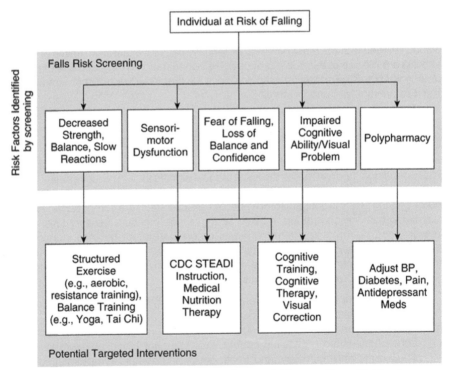

Fig. 2. Link between screening assessments and potential interventions. BP, blood pressure; CDC, Centers for Disease Control and Prevention; STEADI, Stopping Elderly Accidents, Deaths, and Injuries.

from physical activity like faster reaction times, improvements in sensory perception and lower limb strength, and better sympathetic/parasympathetic balance.[17,18,28,81,82] Recent studies have reported that exercise can also lead to improvements in neuropathy symptoms, including increased nerve fiber branching[83] and improved sensory responses in the lower limbs.[84]

SUMMARY

Falls are a major health issue for older adults, especially for those who develop type 2 diabetes who must contend with both age-related declines in balance, muscle strength, and walking ability[7,8,16–18] and health-related issues specific to disease process, including neuropathy, retinopathy, poor glycemic control, electrolyte imbalance, polypharmacy, visual/vestibular problems, cognitive impairment, proprioceptive changes, hypotension, and pain. Given the general association between these variables and falls, being able to identify which measures negatively impact on balance in older diabetic persons is a critical step. Moreover, designing specific interventions to target these physiologic functions underlying balance and gait control will produce the greatest benefit for reducing falls in older persons with diabetes.

REFERENCES

1. Stevens JA, Corso PS, Finkelstein EA, et al. The costs of fatal and non-fatal falls among older adults. Inj Prev 2006;12:290–5.
2. Close JC, Lord SL, Menz HB, et al. What is the role of falls? Best Pract Res Clin Rheumatol 2005;19:913–35.
3. Boyd R, Stevens JA. Falls and fear of falling: burden, beliefs and behaviours. Age Ageing 2009;38:423–8.
4. Lord S, Sherrington C, Menz H, et al. Falls in older people: risk factors and strategies for prevention. Cambridge (United Kingdom): Cambridge University Press; 2007.
5. Pijpers E, Ferreira I, de Jongh RT, et al. Older individuals with diabetes have an increased risk of recurrent falls: analysis of potential mediating factors: the Longitudinal Ageing Study Amsterdam. Age Ageing 2012;41:358–65.
6. Cavanagh PR, Derr JA, Ulbrecht JS, et al. Problems with gait and posture in neuropathic patients with insulin-dependent diabetes mellitus. Diabet Med 1992;9:469–74.
7. Schwartz AV, Hillier TA, Sellmeyer DE, et al. Older women with diabetes have a higher risk of falls: a prospective study. Diabetes Care 2002;25: 1749–54.
8. Schwartz AV, Vittinghoff E, Sellmeyer DE, et al. Diabetes-related complications, glycemic control, and falls in older adults. Diabetes Care 2008;31:391–6.
9. Clark RD, Lord SR, Webster IW. Clinical parameters associated with falls in an elderly population. Gerontology 1993;39:117–23.
10. Lord S, Sherrington C, Menz HB, editors. Falls in older people: risk factors and strategies for prevention. 2nd edition. Cambridge, UK: Cambridge University Press; 2007.
11. Lord SR, Clark RD. Simple physiological and clinical tests for the accurate prediction of falling in older people. Gerontology 1996;42:199–203.
12. Pickering RM, Grimbergen YA, Rigney U, et al. A meta-analysis of six prospective studies of falling in Parkinson's disease. Mov Disord 2007;22: 1892–900.

13. Robinovitch SN, Hsiao ET, Sandler R, et al. Prevention of falls and fall-related fractures through biomechanics. Exerc Sport Sci Rev 2000;28:74–9.
14. Sosnoff J, Motl R, Morrison S. Multiple sclerosis and falls - an evolving tale. US Neurol 2013;9:30–4.
15. Sosnoff JJ, Socie MJ, Boes MK, et al. Mobility, balance and falls in persons with multiple sclerosis. PLoS One 2011;6:e28021.
16. Wallace C, Reiber GE, LeMaster J, et al. Incidence of falls, risk factors for falls, and fall-related fractures in individuals with diabetes and a prior foot ulcer. Diabetes Care 2002;25:1983–6.
17. Morrison S, Colberg SR, Mariano M, et al. Balance training reduces falls risk in older individuals with type 2 diabetes. Diabetes Care 2010;33:748–50.
18. Morrison S, Colberg SR, Parson HK, et al. Relation between risk of falling and postural sway complexity in diabetes. Gait Posture 2012;35:662–8.
19. Richardson JK, Hurvitz EA. Peripheral neuropathy: a true risk factor for falls. J Gerontol A Biol Sci Med Sci 1995;50:M211–5.
20. Berlie HD, Garwood CL. Diabetes medications related to an increased risk of falls and fall-related morbidity in the elderly. Ann Pharmacother 2010;44:712–7.
21. Tilling LM, Darawil K, Britton M. Falls as a complication of diabetes mellitus in older people. J Diabet Complications 2006;20:158–62.
22. Maurer MS, Burcham J, Cheng H. Diabetes mellitus is associated with an increased risk of falls in elderly residents of a long-term care facility. J Gerontol A Biol Sci Med Sci 2005;60:1157–62.
23. Volpato S, Leveille SG, Blaum C, et al. Risk factors for falls in older disabled women with diabetes: the women's health and aging study. J Gerontol A Biol Sci Med Sci 2005;60:1539–45.
24. Volpato S, Maraldi C, Fellin R. Type 2 diabetes and risk for functional decline and disability in older persons. Curr Diabetes Rev 2010;6:134–43.
25. Boucher P, Teasdale N, Courtemanche R, et al. Postural stability in diabetic polyneuropathy. Diabetes Care 1995;18:638–45.
26. Uccioli L, Giacomini PG, Monticone G, et al. Body sway in diabetic neuropathy. Diabetes Care 1995;18:339–44.
27. Witzke KA, Vinik AI. Diabetic neuropathy in older adults. Rev Endocr Metab Disord 2005;6:117–27.
28. Herriott MT, Colberg SR, Parson HK, et al. Effects of 8 weeks of flexibility and resistance training in older adults with type 2 diabetes. Diabetes Care 2004; 27:2988–9.
29. Resnick H, Vinik A, Schwartz A, et al. Independent effects of peripheral nerve dysfunction on lower-extremity physical function in old age. Diabetes Care 2000;23:1642–7.
30. Resnick HE, Stansberry KB, Harris TB, et al. Diabetes, peripheral neuropathy, and old age disability. Muscle Nerve 2002;25:43–50.
31. Strotmeyer ES, de RN, Schwartz AV, et al. The relationship of reduced peripheral nerve function and diabetes with physical performance in older white and black adults: the Health, Aging, and Body Composition (Health ABC) study. Diabetes Care 2008;31:1767–72.
32. Chiles NS, Phillips CL, Volpato S, et al. Diabetes, peripheral neuropathy, and lower-extremity function. J Diabet Complications 2014;28:91–5.
33. Pittenger G, Mehrabyan A, Simmons K, et al. Small fiber neuropathy is associated with the metabolic syndrome. Metab Syndr Relat Disord 2005;3:113–21.
34. Vinik AI, Strotmeyer ES, Nakave AA, et al. Diabetic neuropathy in older adults. Clin Geriatr Med 2008;24:407–35, v.

35. Colberg SR, Parson HK, Nunnold T, et al. Change in cutaneous perfusion following 10 weeks of aerobic training in type 2 diabetes. J Diabet Complications 2005;19: 276–83.
36. Corriveau H, Prince F, Hebert R, et al. Evaluation of postural stability in elderly with diabetic neuropathy. Diabetes Care 2000;23:1187–91.
37. Fioretti S, Scocco M, Ladislao L, et al. Identification of peripheral neuropathy in type-2 diabetic subjects by static posturography and linear discriminant analysis. Gait Posture 2010;32:317–20.
38. Lafond D, Corriveau H, Prince F. Postural control mechanisms during quiet standing in patients with diabetic sensory neuropathy. Diabetes Care 2004;27: 173–8.
39. Lalli P, Chan A, Garven A, et al. Increased gait variability in diabetes mellitus patients with neuropathic pain. J Diabet Complications 2013;27:248–54.
40. Simoneau GG, Ulbrecht J, Derr JA, et al. Postural instability in patients with diabetic sensory neuropathy. Diabetes Care 1994;17:1411–21.
41. Turcot K, Allet L, Golay A, et al. Investigation of standing balance in diabetic patients with and without peripheral neuropathy using accelerometers. Clin Biomech (Bristol, Avon) 2009;24:716–21.
42. Richardson J, Thies S, Ashton-Miller J. An exploration of step time variability on smooth and irregular surfaces in older persons with neuropathy. Clin Biomech 2008;23:349–56.
43. Richardson JK, Thies SB, DeMott TK, et al. Gait analysis in a challenging environment differentiates between fallers and nonfallers among older patients with peripheral neuropathy. Arch Phys Med Rehabil 2005;86:1539–44.
44. Strotmeyer ES, de RN, Schwartz AV, et al. Sensory and motor peripheral nerve function and lower-extremity quadriceps strength: the health, aging and body composition study. J Am Geriatr Soc 2009;57:2004–10.
45. van Dijk PT, Meulenberg OG, van de Sande HJ, et al. Falls in dementia patients. Gerontologist 1993;33:200–4.
46. Coppin AK, Shumway-Cook A, Saczynski JS, et al. Association of executive function and performance of dual-task physical tests among older adults: analyses from the InChianti study. Age Ageing 2006;35:619–24.
47. Hausdorff JM, Yogev G, Springer S, et al. Walking is more like catching than tapping: gait in the elderly as a complex cognitive task. Exp Brain Res 2005; 164:541–8.
48. Imms FJ, Edholm OG. Studies of gait and mobility in the elderly. Age Ageing 1981;10:147–56.
49. Maki BE. Gait changes in older adults: predictors of falls or indicators of fear. J Am Geriatr Soc 1997;45:313–20.
50. Menz HB, Lord SR, Fitzpatrick RC. A structural equation model relating impaired sensorimotor function, fear of falling and gait patterns in older people. Gait Posture 2007;25:243–9.
51. Adkin AL, Frank JS, Carpenter MG, et al. Postural control is scaled to level of postural threat. Gait Posture 2000;12:87–93.
52. Carpenter MG, Frank JS, Silcher CP, et al. The influence of postural threat on the control of upright stance. Exp Brain Res 2001;138:210–8.
53. Delbaere K, Sturnieks DL, Crombez G, et al. Concern about falls elicits changes in gait parameters in conditions of postural threat in older people. J Gerontol A Biol Sci Med Sci 2009;64:237–42.
54. Resnick B. Functional performance of older adults in a long-term care setting. Clin Nurs Res 1998;7:230–46.

55. Vellas BJ, Wayne SJ, Romero LJ, et al. Fear of falling and restriction of mobility in elderly fallers. Age Ageing 1997;26:189–93.
56. Kirkman S, Briscoe V, Clark N, et al. Diabetes in older adults: a consensus report. J Am Geriatr Soc 2012;60:2342.
57. Hanlon JT, Boudreau RM, Roumani YF, et al. Number and dosage of central nervous system medications on recurrent falls in community elders: the Health, Aging and Body Composition study. J Gerontol A Biol Sci Med Sci 2009;64:492–8.
58. Klein BE, Klein R, Knudtson MD, et al. Associations of selected medications and visual function: the Beaver Dam Eye study. Br J Ophthalmol 2003;87:403–8.
59. Woolcott JC, Richardson KJ, Wiens MO, et al. Meta-analysis of the impact of 9 medication classes on falls in elderly persons. Arch Intern Med 2009;169:1952–60.
60. Panel on Prevention of Falls in Older Persons, American Geriatrics Society and British Geriatrics Society. Summary of the updated American Geriatrics Society/British Geriatrics Society clinical practice guideline for prevention of falls in older persons. J Am Geriatr Soc 2011;59:148–57.
61. Lloyd BD, Williamson DA, Singh NA, et al. Recurrent and injurious falls in the year following hip fracture: a prospective study of incidence and risk factors from the Sarcopenia and Hip Fracture study. J Gerontol A Biol Sci Med Sci 2009;64:599–609.
62. American Diabetes Association. Standards of medical care in diabetes. Diabetes Care 2013;36:S11.
63. Ligthelm RJ, Kaiser M, Vora J, et al. Insulin use in elderly adults: risk of hypoglycemia and strategies for care. J Am Geriatr Soc 2012;60:1564–70.
64. Mooradian AD, Perryman K, Fitten J, et al. Cortical function in elderly non-insulin dependent diabetic patients. Behavioral and electrophysiologic studies. Arch Intern Med 1988;148:2369–72.
65. Borenstein J, Aronow HU, Bolton LB, et al. Early recognition of risk factors for adverse outcomes during hospitalization among Medicare patients: a prospective cohort study. BMC Geriatr 2013;13:72.
66. Dyer CA, Taylor GJ, Reed M, et al. Falls prevention in residential care homes: a randomised controlled trial. Age Ageing 2004;33:596–602.
67. Vinik A, Nevoret ML, Casellini C, et al. Diabetic neuropathy. Endocrinol Metab Clin North Am 2013;42:747–87.
68. Renneboog B, Musch W, Vandemergel X, et al. Mild chronic hyponatremia is associated with falls, unsteadiness, and attention deficits. Am J Med 2006;119:71–8.
69. Sandhu HS, Gilles E, DeVita MV, et al. Hyponatremia associated with large-bone fracture in elderly patients. Int Urol Nephrol 2009;41:733–7.
70. Gillespie LD, Robertson MC, Gillespie WJ, et al. Interventions for preventing falls in older people living in the community. Cochrane Database Syst Rev 2009;(2):CD007146.
71. Howe T, Rochester L, Jackson A, et al. Exercise for improving balance in older people. Cochrane Database Syst Rev 2007;2:CD004963.
72. Christmas C, Andersen RA. Exercise and older patients: guidelines for the clinician. J Am Geriatr Soc 2000;48:318–24.
73. Heath JM, Stuart MR. Prescribing exercise for frail elders. J Am Board Fam Pract 2002;15:218–28.
74. Karani R, McLaughlin MA, Cassel CK. Exercise in the healthy older adult. Am J Geriatr Cardiol 2001;10:269–73.

75. Fiatarone MA, O'Neill EF, Ryan ND, et al. Exercise training and nutritional supplementation for physical frailty in very elderly people. N Engl J Med 1994; 330:1769–75.
76. Barnett A, Smith B, Lord SR, et al. Community-based group exercise improves balance and reduces falls in at-risk older people: a randomised controlled trial. Age Ageing 2003;32:407–14.
77. Peterson MJ, Giuliani C, Morey MC, et al. Physical activity as a preventative factor for frailty: the health, aging, and body composition study. J Gerontol A Biol Sci Med Sci 2009;64:61–8.
78. Sherrington C, Lord SR, Herbert RD. A randomised trial of weight-bearing versus non-weight-bearing exercise for improving physical ability in inpatients after hip fracture. Aust J Physiother 2003;49:15–22.
79. Allet L, Armand S, de Bie RA, et al. Clinical factors associated with gait alterations in diabetic patients. Diabet Med 2009;26:1003–9.
80. Allet L, Armand S, de Bie RA, et al. The gait and balance of patients with diabetes can be improved: a randomised controlled trial. Diabetologia 2010; 53:458–66.
81. Colberg S. The impact of exercise on insulin action in type 2 diabetes mellitus: relationship to prevention and control. Insulin 2006;1:85–98.
82. Colberg S, Stansberry K, McNitt P, et al. Chronic exercise is associated with enhanced cutaneous blood flow in type 2 diabetes. J Diabet Complications 2002;16:139–45.
83. Kluding PM, Pasnoor M, Singh R, et al. The effect of exercise on neuropathic symptoms, nerve function, and cutaneous innervation in people with diabetic peripheral neuropathy. J Diabet Complications 2012;26:424–9.
84. Balducci S, Iacobellis G, Parisi L, et al. Exercise training can modify the natural history of diabetic peripheral neuropathy. J Diabet Complications 2006;20: 216–23.

Diabetes and Cognition

Elizabeth Rose Mayeda, PhD, MPH[a],*, Rachel A. Whitmer, PhD[b],
Kristine Yaffe, MD[c,d]

KEYWORDS

- Type 2 diabetes • Cognition • Cognitive decline • Dementia • Aging • Epidemiology

KEY POINTS

- Older adults with type 2 diabetes are 50% to 100% more likely to develop dementia than those without diabetes.
- More research is needed to identify whether the observed association reflects a causal relationship between type 2 diabetes and dementia pathogenesis.
- The proposed link between type 2 diabetes and dementia includes mechanisms contributing to features of Alzheimer's disease and macrovascular and microvascular disorders in the brain.
- Infarcts and atrophy are more common in the brains of older adults with T2D.
- Among people with type 2 diabetes, those with longer duration of diabetes, poorer glycemic control, and more vascular complications are at the highest risk of developing dementia.

INTRODUCTION

Type 2 diabetes (T2D) is highly prevalent among older adults, with more than a quarter of adults age 65 and over in the United States affected by T2D.[1] As the population ages,[2] the prevalence of T2D increases,[3] and the life expectancy for people with T2D extends,[4] understanding the epidemiology of geriatric outcomes, including cognitive decline and dementia, among older adults with T2D is becoming increasingly important. Dementia is a major cause of disability among older adults

Disclosure: The authors were supported by funding from National Institute on Aging grant K24 AG031155, National Institute of Diabetes and Digestive and Kidney Diseases grant R01DK081796, and grant support from the BrightFocus Foundation.
[a] Department of Epidemiology and Biostatistics, University of California, San Francisco, 185 Berry Street, Lobby 5, Suite 5700, San Francisco, CA 94107, USA; [b] Epidemiology, Etiology & Prevention, Kaiser Permanente Division of Research, 2000 Broadway, Oakland, CA 94612, USA; [c] Departments of Psychiatry, Neurology, and Epidemiology and Biostatistics, University of California, San Francisco, Box VAMC - 181, San Francisco, CA 94143, USA; [d] San Francisco Veterans Affairs Medical Center, 4150 Clements St Box VAMC - 181, San Francisco, CA 94121, USA
* Corresponding author.
E-mail address: elizabeth.mayeda@ucsf.edu

and is the fifth leading cause of death for older adults in the United States.[5] Although current pharmacologic treatments for dementia can moderately improve dementia symptoms, no currently available treatment can reverse the neuronal damage or affect disease progression.[6] Understanding the relationship between T2D and dementia could help identify possible strategies for prevention and treatment of dementia.

This article summarizes the existing evidence on the relationship between T2D and dementia. It begins with an overview of dementia and a description of potential mechanisms linking T2D and dementia. Next, it reviews evidence from longitudinal epidemiologic studies examining the relationship between T2D and the incidence of dementia and cognitive decline and evidence from autopsy and brain imaging studies. In addition, risk factors for dementia among older adults with T2D are discussed.

DISEASE DESCRIPTION
Overview of Dementia

Dementia is a syndrome defined as a decline in at least 2 cognitive domains that is severe enough to interfere with daily activities.[7,8] Alzheimer disease and vascular dementia are the two most common causes of dementia, and it is increasingly recognized that most older adults with dementia have features of both Alzheimer disease and cerebrovascular disease.[9–12] In addition to studying dementia, examining the rate of cognitive decline is important for understanding the effects of T2D on cognition among older adults.

Mild cognitive impairment (MCI) is a syndrome of modest cognitive decline that does not interfere with ability to perform activities of daily life and is considered to be a symptomatic predementia state.[13] Not everyone with MCI progresses to dementia, but individuals with MCI develop dementia at higher rates and have a higher mortality than people with normal cognition.[13,14]

Alzheimer Disease and Vascular Dementia

Alzheimer disease and vascular dementia are thought to be the two most common causes of dementia.[6,15] Alzheimer disease is characterized pathologically by neuritic plaques (extracellular deposits of β-amyloid peptides), neurofibrillary tangles (intraneural fibrils of primarily hyperphosphorylated tau protein), loss of synapses and neurons, and brain atrophy.[16] β-Amyloid dysregulation, which leads to plaque formation, is thought to precede synaptic dysfunction and neuronal loss in Alzheimer disease.[9,16] Vascular dementia (also called vascular cognitive impairment) is characterized by macrovascular and microvascular cerebrovascular disease, including clinical stroke and subclinical vascular brain injury.[9]

Diagnosis of Alzheimer disease and vascular dementia in clinical practice are based on objective cognitive assessments, such as neuropsychological testing and history taking from the individual or an informant.[8] Brain autopsy studies have shown that most older people with dementia have features of both Alzheimer disease and cerebrovascular disease[9–12] and that Alzheimer disease features and infarcts are commonly present in the brains of cognitively normal older adults.[10,11,17] These findings suggest that Alzheimer disease, cerebrovascular disease, and cognitive reserve[18] interact in the development of dementia.[9] Because most people with dementia are likely to have mixed pathologies, this article focuses on studies of all-cause dementia, rather than clinically diagnosed Alzheimer disease or vascular dementia.

POTENTIAL MECHANISMS

The interaction between Alzheimer disease, cerebrovascular disease and cognitive reserve[18] in the development of dementia[9] and the complexity of metabolic dysregulation in T2D makes it difficult to identify the mechanisms linking T2D and dementia. The proposed mechanisms include the effects of hyperglycemia and insulin dysregulation (hyperinsulinemia and insulin resistance) on the features of Alzheimer disease and macrovascular and microvascular disease. **Fig. 1** shows the potential mechanisms linking T2D and dementia. It is beyond the scope of this article to cover all possible mechanisms, but this article discusses commonly discussed mechanisms.

Pathophysiology of Type 2 Diabetes

T2D is a complex and heterogeneous metabolic disorder that typically begins with insulin resistance, which is linked to physical inactivity and obesity.[19] In insulin resistance, cells do not use insulin properly, and tissues need more insulin to help glucose enter cells, leading to hyperinsulinemia. Over time, the pancreas loses the ability to secrete enough insulin, and plasma glucose levels increase. It is well established that long-term complications of T2D include microvascular and macrovascular disease throughout the body, including ischemic stroke in the brain.[20] The complexity and heterogeneity of the metabolic dysregulation in T2D and the many years over which it develops and could theoretically have neurologic effects that present a challenge in identifying the neurologic effects of T2D.

Chronic Hyperglycemia

Glucose is the primary source of energy for the brain, but chronic hyperglycemia is known to cause damage to the macrovasculature and microvasculature throughout the body, including ischemic stroke, which can lead to dementia.[15] Retinopathy is a well-established microvascular T2D complication for which there is strong evidence of a causal link with chronic hyperglycemia.[20] Retinal and cerebral arterioles share morphologic and physiologic properties, so retinal microvascular damage is thought to be a marker of cerebral microvascular disease.[21,22] This theory is supported by evidence from epidemiologic studies that have reported that retinopathy is associated with poorer cognitive function,[23] faster cognitive decline,[24] and higher incidence of dementia.[25] This finding supports the hypothesis that chronic hyperglycemia leads to microvascular cerebral damage that can impair cognitive function.

One of the mechanisms through which chronic hyperglycemia damages microvascular tissue is by increasing reactive oxygen species, resulting in oxidative stress.[26] Oxidative damage has also been implicated in the accumulation of β-amyloid and neurofibrillary tangles.[27,28]

Advanced glycation end products (AGEs) are a mechanism through which chronic hyperglycemia contributes to the development of atherosclerosis.[15] AGEs are compounds formed by reactions between proteins, lipids, or nucleic acids and reducing sugars such as glucose that accumulate during aging, but hyperglycemic environments facilitate the creation of AGEs.[29] In addition to contributing to vascular disease, AGEs are found in amyloid plaques and neurofibrillary tangles in people with Alzheimer disease,[30] suggesting that AGEs contribute to Alzheimer disease pathogenesis. The link between AGEs and dementia is further supported by the finding that circulating AGE levels are associated with greater cognitive decline in dementia-free older adults with and without T2D.[31]

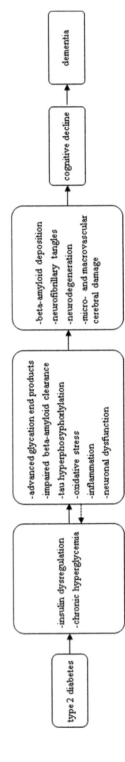

Fig. 1. Potential causal links between type 2 diabetes and cognitive decline and dementia.

Insulin Dysregulation

In addition to cerebral glucose use, insulin has multiple other functions in the brain that support neuronal function, including synaptogenesis, synaptic remodeling, and modulating neurotransmitter levels.[32] Insulin dysregulation includes pathways linked with hyperinsulinemia and functional insulin deficiency in the brain. Insulin dysregulation may impair β-amyloid clearance in the brain and lead to plaque formation by regulating expression of and competing for insulin-degrading enzyme, which degrades β-amyloid in addition to insulin.[33] Additional mechanisms through which insulin dysregulation may lead to Alzheimer disease and cerebrovascular disease include the effects of insulin resistance and hyperinsulinemia on cerebral glucose metabolism, hyperphosphorylation of tau, vascular dysfunction, lipid metabolism, oxidative stress, and inflammation.[32]

Inflammation

Inflammatory mechanisms have also been implicated in pathogenesis of Alzheimer disease[28,34] and vascular dementia.[15] In epidemiologic studies, serum inflammatory markers have been linked with cognitive decline[35] and risk of dementia[36] in older adults. Inflammation has been implicated in development of T2D via contributions to insulin resistance,[37] and insulin dysregulation and chronic hyperglycemia may in turn also promote inflammation.[37]

Noncausal Factors That May Contribute to Association Between Type 2 Diabetes and Dementia

In addition to mechanisms reflecting a causal relationship between T2D and dementia, shared determinants of T2D and dementia may confound the association. Possible confounders include socioeconomic factors, such as educational and occupational attainment; behavioral factors, such as diet and physical activity; and comorbidities, such as obesity and hypertension. Although many studies adjust for these factors, residual confounding may still be present. Reverse causation may also contribute to the observed association between T2D and dementia. Dementia pathogenesis is thought to start to develop decades before manifestation of clinical symptoms,[9] which presents a challenge to establishing temporality, even in longitudinal studies.

EPIDEMIOLOGIC LITERATURE ON TYPE 2 DIABETES AND RISK OF DEMENTIA
Type 2 Diabetes and All-cause Dementia

Table 1 summarizes results from longitudinal epidemiologic studies examining the relationship between T2D and risk of dementia. Estimates of the relative risk (RR) of dementia among people with T2D compared with those without T2D from longitudinal studies range from 1.2 to 2.8, although the confidence intervals (CIs) from some studies include the null. The pooled risk estimate from a recent meta-analysis of 19 longitudinal cohort studies published through 2010 suggested that older adults with T2D have approximately a 50% increased risk of dementia compared with those without T2D (RR, 1.51; 95% CI, 1.31–1.74).[38] More recent studies support an effect size that is at least this large, with risk estimates ranging from 1.6 to 2.4.[39–42]

Because the pathogenesis of dementia is thought to begin many years before the expression of clinical symptoms, examining the relationship between midlife T2D and late-life dementia is of great interest. Three longitudinal cohort studies have examined the relationship between midlife T2D and risk of dementia over a period of 14 to 35 years.[43–45] The association between T2D and incidence of dementia was strong in all 3 studies, which reported hazard ratio estimates ranging from 1.5 to 2.8.

Table 1
Type 2 diabetes and dementia risk among older adults

Publication	Cohort	Baseline Age (y)	Follow-up (y)	N Total	N Diabetes	N Dementia	Diabetes	Dementia Diagnosis	OR or HR (95% CI)
Brayne et al,[84] 1998	Population-based study in Cambridge, United Kingdom	75+	Mean = 2.4	376	17	36	Self-report	Multiphase protocol	OR = 2.6 (0.9–7.8)
Ott et al,[85] 1999	Rotterdam Study, The Netherlands	55+	6	6370	692	126	Medication use, RBS, OGTT	Multiphase protocol	HR = 1.9 (1.3–2.8)
Peila et al,[86] 2002	Honolulu-Asia Aging Study, United States	Mean = 77	Mean = 2.9	2574	900	~130	Self-report, medication use, FBS, OGTT	Multiphase protocol	OR = 1.5 (1.0–2.2)
MacKnight et al,[87] 2002	Canadian Study of Health and Aging, Canada	65+	5	5574	503	467	Self-report, medical records, medication use, RBS	Multiphase protocol	OR = 1.3 (0.9–1.8)
Hassing et al,[88] 2002	Origins of Variance in the Oldest-Old Twin Study, Sweden	80+	6	702	108	187	Self-report, medical records	Multiphase protocol	HR = 1.2 (0.8–1.7)
Schnaider Beeri et al,[43] 2004	Israeli Ischemic Heart Disease Study, Israel	40–65	35	1892	43	309	OGTT, medication use, physician-confirmed diagnosis	Multistep protocol	OR = 2.8 (1.4–5.7)
Whitmer et al,[44] 2005	Data from Kaiser Permanente Northern California, United States	40–44	Mean = 27	8845	1004	721	Self-report, FBS, RBS, medication use	Diagnosis in medical records	HR = 1.5 (1.2–1.8)
Akomolafe et al,[89] 2006	Framingham Study, United States	Mean = 70	20	2210	202	319	RBS, medication use	Multiphase protocol	HR = 1.2 (0.7–2.0)
Irie et al,[90] 2008	Cardiovascular Health Study, United States	65+	8	2547	320	411	FBS, medication use	Multiphase protocol	HR = 1.4 (1.0–2.0)

Study	Age	Years	N			Diabetes ascertainment	Outcome ascertainment	HR (95% CI)
Xu et al,[91] 2009	Kungsholmen Project, Sweden	75+	9	1248	75	420	Diabetes inpatient registry, medication use, RBS	Multiphase protocol	HR = 1.4 (0.9–2.1)
Alonso et al,[45] 2009	Atherosclerosis Risk in Communities Study, United States	46–70	14	11,151	~1445	203	FBS, RBS, self-report, medication use	Hospitalization discharge codes	HR = 2.2 (1.6, 3.0)
Raffaitin et al,[92] 2009	Three-City Study, France	65+	4	7087	~540	208	FBS, RBS, medication use	Multiphase protocol	HR = 1.6 (1.1–2.4)
Ahtiluouto et al,[60] 2010	Vantaa 85+ Study, Finland	85+	10	588	131	106	Self-report, medical record, medication use	Multiphase protocol	HR = 2.1 (1.3–3.3)
Cheng et al,[39] 2011	Washington Heights-Inwood Columbia Aging Project, United States	65+	~9	1488	253	161	Self-report, medication use	Multiphase protocol	HR = 1.7 (1.4–2.9)
Ohara et al,[40] 2011	Hisayama Study, Japan	60+	15	1017	150	232	FBS, OGTT	Multiphase protocol	HR = 1.7 (1.2–2.5)
Kimm et al,[41] 2011	Data from National Health Insurance Corporation, Korea	40–95	14	Women, 358,060 Men, 490,445	Women, ~18,260 Men, ~33,350	Women, 1755 Men, 1497	FBS	Hospitalization discharge codes	Women, HR = 1.6 (1.4–1.9) Men, HR = 1.6 (1.3–1.8)
Mayeda et al,[42] 2013	Sacramento Area Latino Study on Aging, United States	60+	10	1617	677	159	FBS, self-report, medication use	Multiphase protocol; dementia/CIND	Untreated: HR = 1.9 (1.2–3.1) Treated: HR = 2.4 (1.7–3.4)

Abbreviations: CI, confidence interval; CIND, cognitively impaired without dementia; FBS, fasting blood sugar; HR, hazard ratio; OGTT, oral glucose tolerance test; OR, odds ratio; RBS, random blood glucose.

Type 2 Diabetes, Alzheimer Disease, and Vascular Dementia

Several studies have attempted to examine the relationship between T2D, Alzheimer disease, and vascular dementia, rather than all-cause dementia. Overall, there is a stronger association with vascular dementia than Alzheimer disease in the literature. In a recent meta-analysis of 16 studies examining Alzheimer disease and 10 studies examining vascular dementia, the pooled RR for T2D on vascular dementia is larger than the effect size for T2D on Alzheimer disease (vascular dementia, RR 2.48, 95% CI 2.08–2.96; Alzheimer disease, RR 1.46, 95% CI, 1.20–1.77).[38] In addition, the association between T2D and vascular dementia was consistent across studies, and there was considerable variability in the association between T2D and Alzheimer disease. However, these results should be interpreted with caution, because most dementia is thought to be caused by features of both Alzheimer disease and cerebrovascular disease.[9–12]

Type 2 Diabetes and Cognitive Decline

Cross-sectional studies generally report modestly lower cognitive test scores among people with T2D compared with people without T2D. A recent meta-analysis reported median effect sizes of 0.3 to 0.5 standard deviation units across cognitive domains.[46] Evidence relating T2D and cognitive decline is less consistent. Many studies report an association between T2D and decline in 1 or more domains, but across studies there is not a consistent association between T2D and decline in individual domains. One of the most frequently assessed domains in longitudinal studies examining T2D and cognitive change is processing speed: although multiple studies have reported an association between T2D and accelerated decline in processing speed,[47–51] several studies have not found an association.[52–54] T2D and change in memory over time has also been frequently assessed, and although several studies have found an association between T2D and change in memory over time,[49,52,55] some other studies have not.[48,50,56] Evidence is also mixed for change in executive functioning[49,51,56] and verbal fluency.[48,53,55] The inconsistency of results across studies may reflect a weak relationship between T2D and rate of cognitive change or may be due to the cognitive domains assessed, the specific neuropsychological tests used, how rate of cognitive decline was modeled, length of study, or differences in characteristics of study populations.

EVIDENCE FROM NEUROPATHOLOGIC AND NEUROIMAGING STUDIES

Neuropathologic and neuroimaging studies can help elucidate the mechanisms linking T2D and dementia. Most neuropathologic studies have found more infarcts in the brains of people with T2D, but have not found evidence of greater burden of Alzheimer disease (β-amyloid plaques and neurofibrillary tangles), with some studies reporting fewer features of Alzheimer disease in the brains of people with T2D.[57–61] However, in contrast with these findings, evidence from a recent neuropathologic study reported a 2-fold increased risk of autopsy-confirmed Alzheimer disease among older adults with T2D compared with those without T2D.[40]

Neuroimaging studies provide the opportunity to examine brain pathophysiology in vivo, often in larger study samples that are less prone to selection bias than autopsy studies. Structural MRI studies have consistently reported an association between T2D and cortical and subcortical cerebral atrophy among older adults.[56,62–67] Note that cerebral atrophy is not a marker of a specific disease process and can represent neuronal loss from Alzheimer disease or cerebrovascular disease.[68] Thus, although this evidence suggests an effect of T2D on neuronal loss, it does not indicate the specific disease process underlying this change. The association between T2D and cerebral infarcts in structural MRI studies is also consistent across studies.[62–65,67] The association between T2D and white matter hyperintensities, a marker of microvascular cerebral damage, has been inconsistent,[62,64–67] but current structural MRI markers of microvascular disease in the brain may not represent the full spectrum of microvascular damage to the brain that may be relevant for dementia.[69] A recent small study assessed β-amyloid levels using carbon 11–labeled Pittsburgh compound B (PiB) on PET and found no difference in β-amyloid deposition by glucose tolerance (dichotomized as high vs low) or insulin resistance (dichotomized as high vs low).[70]

Taken together, current evidence from neuropathologic and neuroimaging studies suggests that T2D can lead to cerebrovascular damage and brain atrophy, but there is less evidence that T2D leads to Alzheimer disease. More research is needed to better understand the pathologic effects of T2D on the brain.

RISK FACTORS FOR DEMENTIA AMONG PEOPLE WITH TYPE 2 DIABETES

Glycemic control is a central aspect of T2D care and is typically measured by glycosylated hemoglobin A1c (A1c) levels, a measure of the amount of glucose that binds to hemoglobin in red blood cells and represents average glycemic control over several months.[20] Among older adults with T2D, higher A1c levels are associated with lower cognitive function[47,55] and accelerated cognitive decline.[55] Longer duration of T2D and higher A1c levels have been shown to be associated with faster cognitive decline in middle-aged adults with T2D.[49,55] Higher average glucose levels have been shown to be associated with incidence of dementia, not only among older adults with T2D but also among those without T2D.[71]

Severe hypoglycemic events may also contribute to development of dementia in older adults with T2D. Moderate hypoglycemia impairs cognitive function,[72] and severe hypoglycemia may cause neuronal damage.[72,73] Some epidemiologic studies support this hypothesis, because severe hypoglycemic episodes have also been associated with lower cognitive function, faster cognitive decline, and an increased risk of dementia among older adults with T2D.[74–76] However, the relationship between hypoglycemia and dementia may be bidirectional, with hypoglycemic events increasing risk of dementia and impaired cognitive function increasing the risk of hypoglycemic events.[75,76]

Depression and depressive symptoms have been linked with an increased risk of dementia in the general population.[77] Depression is more common among people with T2D than in the general population; it is estimated that nearly 20% of adults with T2D have depression[78] (see the article by Park and colleagues elsewhere in this issue). Two recent studies of members of 2 separate integrated health care delivery systems found that patients with T2D with comorbid depression were twice as likely to develop dementia over 5 years as patients with T2D without depression.[79,80] In the Action to Control Cardiovascular Risk in Diabetes–Memory in Diabetes (ACCORD-MIND) study, participants with depression experienced greater decline in psychomotor speed, verbal memory, and executive function (all domains assessed in this study) over 40 months.[81] Because depression is potentially modifiable, future research is needed to identify whether interventions to treat depression can also reduce cognitive decline in people with T2D.

A 10-year dementia risk score has been developed and validated specifically for older adults with T2D based on 2 large longitudinal cohort studies.[82] This risk score is based on predictors assessable in a primary-care setting and encompasses T2D-specific characteristics. Of the 45 candidate predictors identified from the literature, age, education, microvascular disease, lower extremity complications, cerebrovascular disease, cardiovascular disease, acute metabolic events, and depression were most strongly predictive of dementia. The predictive value of end-organ complications that indicate prolonged exposure to hyperglycemia and cardiovascular risk factors was higher than the predictive value of duration of T2D and A1c levels.

Among people with T2D, some racial/ethnic groups may have a higher risk of dementia. Among older patients with T2D, dementia incidence was 40% to 60% higher among African Americans and Native Americans compared with Asian Americans, and dementia incidence was intermediate among non-Hispanic white and Latino people, even after controlling for sociodemographic factors and clinical characteristics.[83]

SUMMARY

Consistent evidence exists that older adults with T2D are more likely to develop dementia than those without T2D. The literature on the effect of T2D on cognitive decline is less consistent. From a clinical perspective, it is important to know that people with T2D have an increased risk of dementia. However, understanding whether T2D has a causal effect on cognitive decline and dementia and, if so, through what mechanisms is useful for identifying potential strategies to prevent or treat dementia. The biological plausibility of the multiple pathways through which T2D could lead to development of Alzheimer disease and cerebrovascular disease in the brain supports the hypothesis that the link is causal, although current evidence from neuropathologic and neuroimaging studies provides more evidence to support an effect of T2D on cerebrovascular disease than on Alzheimer disease.

Health care providers should be aware that older adults with T2D have an increased risk for development of dementia. Future research is needed to elucidate the pathways linking T2D and dementia, the risk factors for dementia in this high-risk population, and strategies to maintain cognitive function among people with T2D.

REFERENCES

1. Centers for Disease Control and Prevention. National diabetes fact sheet: national estimates and general information on diabetes and prediabetes in the United States, 2011. Available at: http://www.cdc.gov/diabetes/pubs/pdf/ndfs_2011.pdf. Accessed January 24, 2014.
2. Werner CA. The older population: 2010. Washington, DC: US Census Bureau; 2011.
3. Centers for Disease Control and Prevention. Crude and age-adjusted percentage of civilian, noninstitutionalized adults with diagnosed diabetes, United States, 1980–2011. Diabetes data & trends 2013. Available at: http://www.cdc.gov/diabetes/statistics/prev/national/figageadult.htm. Accessed January 13, 2014.
4. Gregg EW, Cheng YJ, Saydah S, et al. Trends in death rates among U.S. adults with and without diabetes between 1997 and 2006: findings from the National Health Interview survey. Diabetes Care 2012;35(6):1252–7.
5. Heron M. Deaths: Leading Causes for 2010. Hyattsville, MD: National Center for Health Statistics; 2013.
6. Thies W, Bleiler L, Alzheimer's Association. 2013 Alzheimer's disease facts and figures. Alzheimers Dement 2013;9(2):208–45.
7. American Psychiatric Association. Diagnostic and statistical manual of mental disorders. 4th edition. Washington, DC: American Psychiatric Publishing; 2000.
8. McKhann GM, Knopman DS, Chertkow H, et al. The diagnosis of dementia due to Alzheimer's disease: recommendations from the National Institute on

Aging-Alzheimer's Association workgroups on diagnostic guidelines for Alzheimer's disease. Alzheimers Dement 2011;7(3):263–9.

9. Jack CR Jr, Knopman DS, Jagust WJ, et al. Tracking pathophysiological processes in Alzheimer's disease: an updated hypothetical model of dynamic biomarkers. Lancet Neurol 2013;12(2):207–16.

10. Schneider JA, Arvanitakis Z, Bang W, Bennett DA. Mixed brain pathologies account for most dementia cases in community-dwelling older persons. Neurology 2007;69(24):2197–204.

11. Brayne C, Richardson K, Matthews FE, et al. Neuropathological correlates of dementia in over-80-year-old brain donors from the population-based Cambridge City Over-75s Cohort (CC75C) study. J Alzheimers Dis 2009;18(3):645–58.

12. Echavarri C, Burgmans S, Caballero MC, et al. Co-occurrence of different pathologies in dementia: implications for dementia diagnosis. J Alzheimers Dis 2012;30(4):909–17.

13. Roberts R, Knopman DS. Classification and epidemiology of MCI. Clin Geriatr Med 2013;29(4):753–72.

14. Campbell NL, Unverzagt F, LaMantia MA, et al. Risk factors for the progression of mild cognitive impairment to dementia. Clin Geriatr Med 2013;29(4):873–93.

15. Gorelick PB, Scuteri A, Black SE, et al. Vascular contributions to cognitive impairment and dementia a statement for healthcare professionals from the American Heart Association/American Stroke Association. Stroke 2011;42(9):2672–713.

16. Weiner MW, Aisen PS, Jack CR Jr, et al. The Alzheimer's disease neuroimaging initiative: progress report and future plans. Alzheimers Dement 2010;6(3):202–11.e7.

17. Bennett DA, Schneider JA, Arvanitakis Z, et al. Neuropathology of older persons without cognitive impairment from two community-based studies. Neurology 2006;66(12):1837–44.

18. Tucker AM, Stern Y. Cognitive reserve in aging. Curr Alzheimer Res 2011;8(4):354–60.

19. Stumvoll M, Goldstein BJ, van Haeften TW. Type 2 diabetes: principles of pathogenesis and therapy. Lancet 2005;365(9467):1333–46.

20. American Diabetes A. Standards of medical care in diabetes–2014. Diabetes Care 2014;37(Suppl 1):S14–80.

21. Patton N, Aslam T, Macgillivray T, et al. Retinal vascular image analysis as a potential screening tool for cerebrovascular disease: a rationale based on homology between cerebral and retinal microvasculatures. J Anat 2005;206(4):319–48.

22. Liew G, Wang JJ, Mitchell P, et al. Retinal vascular imaging: a new tool in microvascular disease research. Circ Cardiovasc Imaging 2008;1(2):156–61.

23. Haan M, Espeland MA, Klein BE, et al. Cognitive function and retinal and ischemic brain changes: the Women's Health Initiative. Neurology 2012;78(13):942–9.

24. Lesage SR, Mosley TH, Wong TY, et al. Retinal microvascular abnormalities and cognitive decline: the ARIC 14-year follow-up study. Neurology 2009;73(11):862–8.

25. Exalto LG, Biessels GJ, Karter AJ, et al. Severe diabetic retinal microvascular eye disease and dementia risk in type 2 diabetes. J Alzheimers Dis 2014;42(0):S109–17.

26. Ceriello A, Taboga C, Tonutti L, et al. Evidence for an independent and cumulative effect of postprandial hypertriglyceridemia and hyperglycemia on

endothelial dysfunction and oxidative stress generation: effects of short- and long-term simvastatin treatment. Circulation 2002;106(10):1211–8.

27. Nunomura A, Perry G, Aliev G, et al. Oxidative damage is the earliest event in Alzheimer disease. J Neuropathol Exp Neurol 2001;60(8):759–67.

28. Galasko D, Montine TJ. Biomarkers of oxidative damage and inflammation in Alzheimer's disease. Biomark Med 2010;4(1):27–36.

29. Goldin A, Beckman JA, Schmidt AM, et al. Advanced glycation end products sparking the development of diabetic vascular injury. Circulation 2006;114(6): 597–605.

30. Srikanth V, Maczurek A, Phan T, et al. Advanced glycation endproducts and their receptor RAGE in Alzheimer's disease. Neurobiol Aging 2011;32(5):763–77.

31. Yaffe K, Lindquist K, Schwartz AV, et al. Advanced glycation end product level diabetes, and accelerated cognitive aging. Neurology 2011;77(14):1351–6.

32. Craft S, Cholerton B, Baker LD. Insulin and Alzheimer's disease: untangling the web. J Alzheimers Dis 2013;33(Suppl 1):S263–75.

33. Craft S. The role of insulin dysregulation in aging and Alzheimer's disease. In: Craft S, Christen Y, editors. Diabetes, insulin and Alzheimer's disease. Berlin: Springer-Verlag Berlin Heidelberg; 2010. p. 109–27.

34. Akiyama H, Barger S, Barnum S, et al. Inflammation and Alzheimer's disease. Neurobiol Aging 2000;21(3):383–421.

35. Yaffe K, Lindquist K, Penninx BW, et al. Inflammatory markers and cognition in well-functioning African-American and white elders. Neurology 2003;61(1): 76–80.

36. Schmidt R, Schmidt H, Curb JD, et al. Early inflammation and dementia: a 25-year follow-up of the Honolulu-Asia Aging Study. Ann Neurol 2002;52(2):168–74.

37. Dandona P, Aljada A, Bandyopadhyay A. Inflammation: the link between insulin resistance, obesity and diabetes. Trends Immunol 2004;25(1):4–7.

38. Cheng G, Huang C, Deng H, et al. Diabetes as a risk factor for dementia and mild cognitive impairment: a meta-analysis of longitudinal studies. Intern Med J 2012;42(5):484–91.

39. Cheng D, Noble J, Tang MX, et al. Type 2 diabetes and late-onset Alzheimer's disease. Dement Geriatr Cogn Disord 2011;31(6):424–30.

40. Ohara T, Doi Y, Ninomiya T, et al. Glucose tolerance status and risk of dementia in the community: the Hisayama Study. Neurology 2011;77(12):1126–34.

41. Kimm H, Lee PH, Shin YJ, et al. Mid-life and late-life vascular risk factors and dementia in Korean men and women. Arch Gerontol Geriatr 2011;52(3): e117–22.

42. Mayeda ER, Haan MN, Kanaya AK, et al. Type 2 diabetes and 10 year risk of dementia and cognitive impairment among older Mexican Americans. Diabetes Care 2013;36(9):2600–6.

43. Schnaider Beeri M, Goldbourt U, Silverman JM, et al. Diabetes mellitus in midlife and the risk of dementia three decades later. Neurology 2004;63(10):1902–7.

44. Whitmer RA, Sidney S, Selby J, et al. Midlife cardiovascular risk factors and risk of dementia in late life. Neurology 2005;64(2):277–81.

45. Alonso A, Mosley TH Jr, Gottesman RF, et al. Risk of dementia hospitalisation associated with cardiovascular risk factors in midlife and older age: the Atherosclerosis Risk in Communities (ARIC) study. J Neurol Neurosurg Psychiatr 2009; 80(11):1194–201.

46. van den Berg E, Kloppenborg RP, Kessels RP, et al. Type 2 diabetes mellitus, hypertension, dyslipidemia and obesity: a systematic comparison of their impact on cognition. Biochim Biophys Acta 2009;1792(5):470–81.

47. Yaffe K, Falvey C, Hamilton N, et al. Diabetes, glucose control, and 9-year cognitive decline among older adults without dementia. Arch Neurol 2012;69(9): 1170–5.
48. Knopman DS, Mosley TH, Catellier DJ, et al. Fourteen-year longitudinal study of vascular risk factors, *APOE* genotype, and cognition: the ARIC MRI Study. Alzheimers Dement 2009;5(3):207–14.
49. Spauwen PJ, Köhler S, Verhey FR, et al. Effects of type 2 diabetes on 12-year cognitive change: results from the Maastricht Aging Study. Diabetes Care 2013;36(6):1554–61.
50. Arvanitakis Z, Wilson RS, Bienias JL, et al. Diabetes mellitus and risk of Alzheimer disease and decline in cognitive function. Arch Neurol 2004;61(5):661–6.
51. Gregg EW, Yaffe K, Cauley JA, et al. Is diabetes associated with cognitive impairment and cognitive decline among older women? Study of Osteoporotic Fractures Research Group. Arch Intern Med 2000;160(2):174–80.
52. Comijs HC, Kriegsman DM, Dik MG, et al. Somatic chronic diseases and 6-year change in cognitive functioning among older persons. Arch Gerontol Geriatr 2009;48(2):191–6.
53. Van den Berg E, De Craen A, Biessels G, et al. The impact of diabetes mellitus on cognitive decline in the oldest of the old: a prospective population-based study. Diabetologia 2006;49(9):2015–23.
54. Nooyens AC, Baan CA, Spijkerman AM, et al. Type 2 diabetes and cognitive decline in middle-aged men and women: the Doetinchem Cohort Study. Diabetes Care 2010;33(9):1964–9.
55. Tuligenga RH, Dugravot A, Tabák AG, et al. Midlife type 2 diabetes and poor glycaemic control as risk factors for cognitive decline in early old age: a post-hoc analysis of the Whitehall II cohort study. Lancet Diabetes Endocrinol 2014;2(3):228–35.
56. Debette S, Seshadri S, Beiser A, et al. Midlife vascular risk factor exposure accelerates structural brain aging and cognitive decline. Neurology 2011;77(5):461–8.
57. Heitner J, Dickson D. Diabetics do not have increased Alzheimer-type pathology compared with age-matched control subjects. A retrospective postmortem immunocytochemical and histofluorescent study. Neurology 1997;49(5): 1306–11.
58. Janson J, Laedtke T, Parisi JE, et al. Increased risk of type 2 diabetes in Alzheimer disease. Diabetes 2004;53(2):474–81.
59. Alafuzoff I, Aho L, Helisalmi S, et al. Beta-amyloid deposition in brains of subjects with diabetes. Neuropathol Appl Neurobiol 2009;35(1):60–8.
60. Ahtiluoto S, Polvikoski T, Peltonen M, et al. Diabetes, Alzheimer disease, and vascular dementia: a population-based neuropathologic study. Neurology 2010;75(13):1195–202.
61. Beeri MS, Silverman JM, Davis KL, et al. Type 2 diabetes is negatively associated with Alzheimer's disease neuropathology. J Gerontol A Biol Sci Med Sci 2005;60(4):471–5.
62. Manschot SM, Brands AM, van der Grond J, et al. Brain magnetic resonance imaging correlates of impaired cognition in patients with type 2 diabetes. Diabetes 2006;55(4):1106–13.
63. Espeland MA, Bryan RN, Goveas JS, et al. Influence of type 2 diabetes on brain volumes and changes in brain volumes: results from the Women's Health Initiative magnetic resonance imaging studies. Diabetes Care 2013;36(1):90–7.
64. Moran C, Phan TG, Chen J, et al. Brain atrophy in type 2 diabetes: regional distribution and influence on cognition. Diabetes Care 2013;36(12):4036–42.

65. van Harten B, de Leeuw FE, Weinstein HC, et al. Brain imaging in patients with diabetes a systematic review. Diabetes Care 2006;29(11):2539–48.
66. Falvey CM, Rosano C, Simonsick EM, et al. Macro-and microstructural magnetic resonance imaging indices associated with diabetes among community-dwelling older adults. Diabetes Care 2013;36(3):677–82.
67. Saczynski JS, Siggurdsson S, Jonsson PV, et al. Glycemic status and brain injury in older individuals: the age gene/environment susceptibility–Reykjavik Study. Diabetes Care 2009;32(9):1608–13.
68. Jack CR Jr. Alliance for aging research AD biomarkers work group: structural MRI. Neurobiol Aging 2011;32(Suppl 1):S48–57.
69. Pantoni L. Cerebral small vessel disease: from pathogenesis and clinical characteristics to therapeutic challenges. Lancet Neurol 2010;9(7):689–701.
70. Thambisetty M, Jeffrey Metter E, Yang A, et al. Glucose intolerance, insulin resistance, and pathological features of Alzheimer disease in the Baltimore Longitudinal Study of Aging. JAMA Neurol 2013;70(9):1167–72.
71. Crane PK, Walker R, Hubbard RA, et al. Glucose levels and risk of dementia. N Engl J Med 2013;369(6):540–8.
72. Warren RE, Frier BM. Hypoglycaemia and cognitive function. Diabetes Obes Metab 2005;7(5):493–503.
73. Bree AJ, Puente EC, Daphna-Iken D, et al. Diabetes increases brain damage caused by severe hypoglycemia. Am J Physiol Endocrinol Metab 2009; 297(1):E194–201.
74. Whitmer RA, Karter AJ, Yaffe K, et al. Hypoglycemic episodes and risk of dementia in older patients with type 2 diabetes mellitus. JAMA 2009;301(15): 1565–72.
75. Feinkohl I, Aung PP, Keller M, et al. Severe hypoglycemia and cognitive decline in older people with type 2 diabetes: the Edinburgh Type 2 Diabetes Study. Diabetes Care 2014;37(2):507–15.
76. Yaffe K, Falvey CM, Hamilton N, et al. Association between hypoglycemia and dementia in a biracial cohort of older adults with diabetes mellitus. JAMA Intern Med 2013;173(14):1300–6.
77. Byers AL, Yaffe K. Depression and risk of developing dementia. Nat Rev Neurol 2011;7(6):323–31.
78. Ali S, Stone MA, Peters JL, et al. The prevalence of co-morbid depression in adults with type 2 diabetes: a systematic review and meta-analysis. Diabet Med 2006;23(11):1165–73.
79. Katon W, Lyles CR, Parker MM, et al. Association of depression with increased risk of dementia in patients with type 2 diabetes: the Diabetes and Aging Study. Arch Gen Psychiatry 2012;69(4):410–7.
80. Katon WJ, Lin EH, Williams LH, et al. Comorbid depression is associated with an increased risk of dementia diagnosis in patients with diabetes: a prospective cohort study. J Gen Intern Med 2010;25(5):423–9.
81. Sullivan MD, Katon WJ, Lovato LC, et al. Association of depression with accelerated cognitive decline among patients with type 2 diabetes in the ACCORD-MIND trial. JAMA Psychiatry 2013;70(10):1041–7.
82. Exalto LG, Biessels GJ, Karter AJ, et al. Risk score for prediction of 10 year dementia risk in individuals with type 2 diabetes: a cohort study. Lancet Diabetes Endocrinol 2013;1(3):183–90.
83. Mayeda ER, Karter AJ, Huang ES, et al. Racial/ethnic differences in dementia risk among older type 2 diabetes patients: the Diabetes and Aging Study. Diabetes Care 2014;37(4):1009–15.

84. Brayne C, Gill C, Huppert FA, et al. Vascular risks and incident dementia: results from a cohort study of the very old. Dement Geriatr Cogn Disord 1998;9(3): 175–80.
85. Ott A, Stolk RP, van Harskamp F, et al. Diabetes mellitus and the risk of dementia: the Rotterdam Study. Neurology 1999;53(9):1937–42.
86. Peila R, Rodriguez BL, Launer LJ. Type 2 diabetes, APOE gene, and the risk for dementia and related pathologies: the Honolulu-Asia Aging Study. Diabetes 2002;51(4):1256–62.
87. MacKnight C, Rockwood K, Awalt E, et al. Diabetes mellitus and the risk of dementia, Alzheimer's disease and vascular cognitive impairment in the Canadian Study of Health and Aging. Dement Geriatr Cogn Disord 2002;14(2):77–83.
88. Hassing LB, Johansson B, Nilsson SE, et al. Diabetes mellitus is a risk factor for vascular dementia, but not for Alzheimer's disease: a population-based study of the oldest old. Int Psychogeriatr 2002;14(3):239–48.
89. Akomolafe A, Beiser A, Meigs JB, et al. Diabetes mellitus and risk of developing Alzheimer disease: results from the Framingham Study. Arch Neurol 2006; 63(11):1551–5.
90. Irie F, Fitzpatrick AL, Lopez OL, et al. Enhanced risk for Alzheimer disease in persons with type 2 diabetes and APOE epsilon4: the Cardiovascular Health Study Cognition Study. Arch Neurol 2008;65(1):89–93.
91. Xu WL, von Strauss E, Qiu CX, et al. Uncontrolled diabetes increases the risk of Alzheimer's disease: a population-based cohort study. Diabetologia 2009;52(6): 1031–9.
92. Raffaitin C, Gin H, Empana JP, et al. Metabolic syndrome and risk for incident Alzheimer's disease or vascular dementia: the Three-City Study. Diabetes Care 2009;32(1):169–74.

Depression Among Older Adults with Diabetes Mellitus

 CrossMark

Mijung Park, PhD, MPH, RN[a],*, Charles F. Reynolds III, MD[b]

KEYWORDS

- Diabetes • Depression • Mood disorders • Aging • Collaborative care

KEY POINTS

- Depression is highly prevalent in the general population and increases the risk for type 2 diabetes mellitus (DM).
- Comorbid depression and DM are associated with negative health outcomes, such as accelerated cognitive decline and increased mortality.
- Depression impinges the patient and the family caregiver's ability to effectively manage DM, decreases adherence to treatment, and undermines the successful physician-patient relationship.
- Effective models for treating comorbid depression and DM exist, and some components of these models are implementable in individual clinics.

INTRODUCTION

Diabetes mellitus (DM) is one of the most common chronic conditions among older adults. About 26.9%, or 10.9 million, US residents aged 65 years and older had diabetes in 2010.[1] Depressive disorders are serious chronic diseases that increase morbidity and mortality,[2] erode quality of life,[3] and increase medical expenditure.[4–8] Depression and DM often co-occur. Data from a range of settings suggest that the prognosis of both DM and depression, in terms of severity of disease, complications, treatment resistance, and mortality, is worse for either disease when they are comorbid than when they occur separately. Comorbid depression in patients with DM is strongly associated with increased burdens of DM symptoms,[9] poor self-management and treatment adherence,[10] increased health care services utilization

[a] Department of Health and Community Systems, University of Pittsburgh, School of Nursing, 3500 Victoria Street, 421 Victoria Building, Pittsburgh, PA 15213, USA; [b] NIMH Center of Excellence in Late Life Depression Prevention and Treatment, Hartford Center of Excellence in Geriatric Psychiatry, Aging Institute of UPMC Senior Services and University of Pittsburgh, 3811 O'Hara Street, Pittsburgh, PA 15213-2582, USA
* Corresponding author.
E-mail address: parkm@pitt.edu

Clin Geriatr Med 31 (2015) 117–137
http://dx.doi.org/10.1016/j.cger.2014.08.022
0749-0690/15/$ – see front matter © 2015 Elsevier Inc. All rights reserved.
geriatric.theclinics.com

and medical expenditures,[11] and an increased risk of DM complications.[12] DM complications, such as myocardial infarction, amputation, or loss of vision, can in turn precipitate or worsen depressive episodes. Nevertheless, few studies have extensively examined the associations between depression and DM in the older adult population. Also, recent studies have found that the combination of DM and depression may increase the risk for dementia, suggesting increased brain toxicity.[13] The purpose of this review is to summarize the clinical presentation of late-life depression among older adults with DM, potential mechanisms of comorbidity of depression and DM, importance of depression in the successful management of DM, and available best practice models for depression treatment.

DISEASE DESCRIPTION

Depression is a mood disorder that causes a persistent feeling of sadness and loss of interest. To be diagnosed with major depression, a patient must have depressed mood or anhedonia and at least 5 of the following 9 symptoms nearly every day for at least 2 weeks:

- Depressed mood
- Marked diminished interest/pleasure
- Sleep disturbance (increased or decreased sleep)
- Appetite disturbance (increased or decreased appetite; typically with weight change)
- Fatigue/loss or energy
- Diminished concentration or indecisiveness
- Feelings of worthlessness or excessive or inappropriate guilt
- Psychomotor retardation or agitation (a change in mental and physical speed perceived by other people)
- Recurrent thoughts of death or suicide (not just fear of dying)

They must also experience functional impairment related to these depressive symptoms.

Older adults, however, do not always present with the typical symptoms of depression. In particular, depressed or sad mood may be less evident or not even present. In these cases, anhedonia may be a better indicator for depression.[14,15] Depressed older adults may experience sleep disturbances (sleeping too much or too little) or changes in appetite (eating too much or too little). Decrease in self-efficacy, motivation, and ability to participate in self-care may also indicate underlying depressive symptoms. Signs of such symptoms can be subtle. Older adults may reply with "I don't know" to simple questions, decline to participate in physical, speech, or occupational therapy, and feel negative or hopeless about treatments offered. Some may easily give up tasks during these therapies. Older adults who experience loss of self-worth or sense of loneliness due to depression may complain "nobody needs me" or "I feel I am just in everyone's way." The symptoms of late-life depression are often attributed to normal aging, grief, physical illness, or dementia and providers and patients miss important opportunities to initiate treatment for what is a treatable health problem.[16]

Most older adults with clinically significant depressive symptoms do not meet standard diagnostic criteria for major depression or dysthymic disorder.[17,18] Patients in this group fall short of meeting diagnostic criteria for major depression because of fewer or limited duration of depression symptoms. Nonetheless, studies suggest that these patients carry similar disease burden: poorer health outcomes, functional impairment, and higher health utilization and treatment costs.[19-21] Moreover, these patients are at very high risk for subsequently developing major depression and may also develop suicidal ideation.[22–24]

Although depression can be successfully treated,[25] many older adults suffer from chronic or recurrent depression.[26] In a prospective study about courses of major depression, approximately 85% of individuals who recover from depression experience recurrence within 15 years.[27] Findings of meta-analyses of chronic depression in primary care and community samples suggest that about 1 in 3 depressed older adults experience chronic and persistent course.[28,29] Depressed patients with DM are at greater risk for a chronic course of depression or less complete recovery.[30] Such chronicity, in turn, makes it more difficult for older adults and their family caregivers to optimally self-manage DM.

In the older adults with DM, depressive symptoms may be overlooked because they are assumed to be due to concurrent DM and other medical illnesses. Many of the symptoms of depression, such as lower energy, fatigue, loss of appetite, and sleep disturbance, are also associated with DM. Thus, differentiating stress related to DM self-management and depression can be challenging.[31] Somatic complaints may suggest the presence of depression, especially if they are out of proportion to underlying physical disorders.[32] Only 25% to 30% of primary care patients present with purely affective or cognitive symptoms of depression.[33]

RISK FACTORS

Risk factors for developing depression after age 65 are similar to those in younger individuals and include being female gender, being unmarried, being of low socioeconomic status, or having chronic physical illness, social isolation, a history of depression, or a family history of depression. The risk of major depression increases up to 3-fold if a first-degree relative has the illness.[34] Additional risk factors that are particularly important in older adults include loss and grief,[35] social isolation or limited social support,[36] high degrees of family conflict,[37,38] and care-taking responsibilities.[39] Other risk factors that increase the likelihood of depression in the medically ill elderly include the presence of cognitive impairment, age greater than 75, active alcohol abuse, and lower educational attainment.[40–47] **Table 1** summarized the risk factors for depression in older adults.

PROTECTIVE FACTORS

Strong and supportive social context has been identified as a protective factor. A compelling body of evidence has shown that social support decreases the risks for depression[48,49] and for depression relapse,[50] increases adherence to depression treatment,[51,52] and improves treatment outcomes. Social support may have positive effects on psychological well-being independent of whether or not individuals are exposed to stress.[53,54] Social support may also promote well-being through modulation of neuro-endocrine response to stress.[55]

Social activities, such as volunteering, are suggested to have a positive effect on depression outcomes in older adults.[56] Studies have also suggested that religion and spirituality may play an important part in many older adults' lives, and social connectedness and support are an important part of organized religion.[57] Religion may allow older adults to experience life as meaningful despite losses and challenges and, thereby, reduce the risk of depression. It is also possible that the positive effect of religion on mental health is mediated by the social connectedness and the social support derived from taking part in religious activities.

Table 1
Risk factors for depression in older adults

Authors, Year	Sample	Finding
Age		
Cole & Dendukuri,[150] 2003	Age ≥50	Meta-analysis of epidemiologic studies. Pooled OR for depression associated with age: 1.2 (95% CI: 0.9–1.7)
Snowden,[151] 2001	Mixed age	Comprehensive review of epidemiologic studies: depression is as common in older age as in earlier life
Being female		
Cole & Dendukuri,[150] 2003	Age ≥50	Meta-analysis of epidemiologic studies. Pooled OR for depression associated with being female: 1.4 (95% CI: 1.2–1.8)
Sonnenberg et al,[152] 2000	Age 55 to ≤85	A random, age-stratified and sex-stratified community sample of 3056 older Dutch people; prevalence of depression in women was almost twice as high as in men
Grief and loss		
Zisook & Shuchter,[153] 1991	Mixed age	Major depression and anxiety disorders are common within the first year of the spouse's death: 29%–58% meet criteria for major depression at 1 mo, 24%–30% at 2 mo, and 25% at 3 mo
Cole & Dendukuri,[150] 2003	Age ≥50	Meta-analysis of epidemiologic studies. Pooled OR for depression associated with recent bereavement: 3.3 (95% CI: 1.7–4.9)
Turvey et al,[154] 1999	Age ≥70	The rate of syndromal depression in the newly bereaved was nearly 9 times as high as the rate for married individuals, and the rate of depressive symptoms was nearly 4 times as high
Social isolation		
Cole & Dendukuri,[150] 2003	Age ≥50	Meta-analysis of epidemiologic studies. Pooled OR for depression associated with living alone: 1.7 (95% CI: 0.6–4.7)
Prince et al,[155] 1998	Age ≥65	Prospective epidemiologic study. Lack of contact with friends was a direct risk factor but also modified the association between handicap and depression
Cacioppo et al,[156] 2006	Age ≥55	There is a reciprocal relationship between loneliness depressive symptoms and time
Cognitive impairment		
Cole & Dendukuri,[150] 2003	Age ≥50	Meta-analysis of epidemiologic studies. Pooled OR for depression associated with recent bereavement: 2.1 (95% CI: 0.6–8.6)

PREVALENCE/INCIDENCE

Depression is one of the most common mental disorders in late life.[58] About 1 in 4 US residents is projected to experience major depression by age 75.[59] In community settings, about 5% of adults aged 65 and older meet research diagnostic criteria for major depression,[60,61] with rates of subsyndromal, clinically significant depression estimated at 8% to 16%.[62] The rates of geriatric depression increase to 12% to 30% in institutional settings, and up to 50% for residents in long-term care facilities.[63,64] Approximately 5% to 10% of older adults seen in primary care settings have clinically significant depression.[65]

Variations in prevalence in late-life depression across racial/ethnic groups are rarely examined and existing literature presents mixed findings. However, given that differences in diabetes prevalence exist by racial/ethnic group, these may be important to appreciate. A cross-sectional and longitudinal epidemiologic study showed that non-Hispanic white and Latino older adults have higher rates of depression.[66–68] A longitudinal population study of community-dwelling Hispanic older adults showed approximately 9% of the sample met the criteria for lifetime diagnosis of major depression, whereas 24% of the sample reported minor depression.[68] The prevalence of depression in African Americans is generally lower than their white counterparts.[69]

Minority older adults are less likely to be diagnosed with or treated for depression than their white counterparts.[70,71] These health service disparities in minority populations become increasingly complicated when considering cultural beliefs and attitudes toward depression care. Culture influences how individuals experience and express depression.[72,73] Minority patients from certain ethnic groups may express their depression more somatically than psychologically.[33,74] Such somatic presentations may reduce the recognition of depression by primary care providers or lead to the perception of a patient as "difficult."[75] Some minorities may also have less faith in the biological cause of depression, be more skeptical about antidepressant use, and show stronger preferences for counseling than their white counterparts.[76,77] When pharmaceutical treatment is the only available option, minority older adults may be less likely to engage in treatment and more likely to be nonadherent. The present primary care systems that focus primarily on pharmacologic treatment without considering the unique barriers faced by ethnic and racial minority populations may not affect the pattern of disparities observed.[78]

Scant information on the cross-national prevalence of late-life depression is available. A report from the World Health Organization concluded that older adults in developed countries had relatively low average depression rates of 2.6%, whereas those in developing countries had an average rate almost 3 times higher (7.5%).[79] The rapid increase in diabetes across the world, particularly in developing countries,[80,81] indicates that these international discrepancies are critical to understand.

Among older adults with DM, depression is highly prevalent.[82] Up to 30% of individuals with DM have a significant number of depressive symptoms and 12% to 18% meet diagnostic criteria for major depression.[3,83] Patients with DM experience significantly higher rates of depression compared with their age-matched and gender-matched counterparts.[82] A meta-analysis of 10 studies showed that the prevalence of depression was significantly higher in patients with DM compared with those without DM (17.6 vs 9.8%).[82] The prevalence of depression was higher in women with diabetes (23.8%) compared with men with diabetes (12.8%); however, the odds ratio (OR) for depression in patients with type 2 DM compared with those without was higher in men (OR = 1.9, 95% confidence interval [CI] 1.7–2.1) than women (OR = 1.3, 95% CI 1.2–1.4).

DEPRESSION AND MORTALITY IN INDIVIDUALS WITH DIABETES MELLITUS

Based on several meta-analyses, depression is associated with a 1.5-fold to 2.6-fold increase of mortality among individuals with DM.[7,84,85] Few studies have examined if treating depression may decrease mortality among individuals with depression. Data from a large clinical trial of a collaborative late-life depression treatment program in the primary care setting (PROSPECT) showed that evidence-based treatment of depression can reduce rates of mortality among those with DM (adjusted hazard ratio 0.49, 95% CI: 0.24–0.98).[86] Another study of all-cause mortality with the same sample also found that patients with major depression in intervention practice were 24% less likely to have died, compared with depressed older adults in usual primary care practices.[87]

UNDERLYING MECHANISMS OF COMORBIDITY OF DEPRESSION AND DIABETES MELLITUS

Katon[88] proposed a complex bidirectional relationship between depression and type 2 DM (**Fig. 1**). Depression early in adult life is a risk factor for subsequent development of DM.[89] The increased risk of DM in patients with depression has been hypothesized to be the result of maladaptive health risk behaviors associated with depression, such as smoking, obesity, and lack of physical exercise,[88] as well as psychobiologic factors, such as increased cortisol levels, increased inflammatory factors,[90] and insulin resistance.[91]

On the other hand, DM may increase the risk of depression or worsen the depression symptoms because of increased symptom burden, DM complications causing functional impairment, and decreased quality of life, as well as vascular brain changes secondary to DM. Comorbid depression has been found to impair the ability to perform self-care activities necessary to control DM by affecting memory, energy level, and executive function.[92–94] Lack of self-care and the psychobiologic changes associated with comorbid depression may explain why individuals with comorbid depression experience increased risk of macrovascular and microvascular complications[12] and dementia.[13]

Although DM and depression are independently associated with memory and cognitive impairment,[95–97] recent clinical epidemiologic studies found that concurrent DM and depression may have a synergistic negative effect on brain health, posing greater risk for developing dementia and Alzheimer disease.[13] There are several biological mechanisms that can explain such a toxic effect of the DM and depression combination on brain health. First, DM and depression are risk factors for cardiovascular and cerebrovascular diseases (eg, vascular dementia and Alzheimer disease). Concurrent DM and depression may increase risk for cardiovascular and cerebrovascular events in additive fashion.[13] Second, depression is associated with dysregulation of the hypothalamic-pituitary axis,[98,99] which increases glucocorticoid production and impairs negative feedback. Hypercortisolemia is associated with metabolic syndrome, a risk factor for vascular dementia and Alzheimer disease.[100–102] Finally, chronic or recurrent depression is associated with hippocampal atrophy.[103,104]

The temporal relationship between depression and DM has not been fully established. Existing evidence suggests that the association between history of depression and subsequent development of DM is stronger than that between the history of DM and the subsequent development of depression.[105] Several prospective epidemiologic studies have found that having depression increased the risk for developing DM in subsequent years by 1.62-fold to 2.52-fold: Demakakos and colleagues[106]

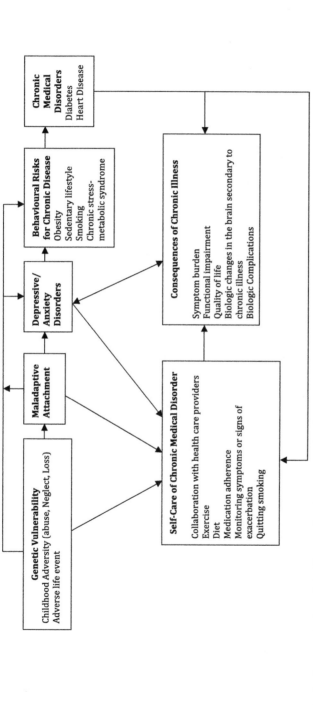

Fig. 1. A conceptual model of interaction between major depression and medical illness. (*Reproduced from Katon WJ. Clinical and health services relationships between major depression, depressive symptoms, and general medical illness. Biol Psychiatry 2003;54(3):216–26.*)

analyzed data of 6111 individuals who reported not having doctor-diagnosed DM at baseline in 2002 to 2003 and concluded that, after adjusting for several demographic and clinical characteristics, individuals who had greater depressive symptoms at baseline experienced a 1.62-fold increased risk for developing DM in the subsequent 45.8 months. In another longitudinal study of a community-residing adult population by Carnethon and colleagues,[107] after adjusting for age, race, and gender, the adjusted risk of developing DM in subsequent years are 2.52-fold higher among those with greater depressive symptoms than those with low depressive symptoms. A prospective epidemiologic study of 1715 residents of the Baltimore Catchment area showed that having a major depressive disorder was associated with a more than 2-fold increase in risk (adjusted OR: 2.23; 95% CI 0.90–5.55) for developing DM in the subsequent 13 years.[108] However, this was not statistically significant.

Having DM increases the risk for subsequently developing depression. A meta-analysis of 11 epidemiologic studies concluded that individuals who had type 2 DM without depression at baseline experienced a 1.24-fold increased risk (95% CI 1.09–1.40) for subsequently developing or recurring depression in subsequent years.[109] Data from the study of 5201 multiracial participants of the Women's Health Across the Nation concluded that having DM increase the odds for developing DM in the subsequent 2 years by 2.8-fold (95% CI: 1.2–6.4) among depressed African American women.[89] Therefore, older adults with diabetes should be considered at higher risk for future depression.

PREVENTION AND EARLY TREATMENT

Prevention and early treatment of depression matter to providers who treat individuals with DM for several reasons. First, as mentioned earlier, having depression may increase the risk for subsequently developing DM. Thus, prevention and early treatment of depression may lower the incidence of DM. Second, having comorbid depression decreases the individual's ability to successfully self-manage DM and increases the likelihood for poor DM outcomes. Third, depression is treatable and several treatment approaches are developed for primary care settings. A recent clinical trial with 247 older adults[110] suggests that both problem-solving therapy for primary care and coaching in health dietary practices could effectively reduce the incidence of major depression in older adults, including in older African American adults with high body mass index. Despite that African American participants in the trial carried a greater risk for depression than did their white counterparts, including obesity, the interventions were equally effective in reducing the incidence of major depression from an expected rate of 20% to 25% over a period of 2 years to only 8% to 9%, in both African American older adults and white older adults. Thus, given the challenges of treating prevalent depression in people living with both depression and DM, especially in minority populations, where stigma represents an important barrier, it seems particularly important to develop depression prevention strategies that use, variously, active coping strategies and lifestyle interventions that promote health and protective factors.

The US Preventive Services Task Force found at least fair evidence that screening adults for depression improves health outcomes and that benefits outweigh harms (B rating) and recommends screening for depression if practices have systems in place to assure accurate diagnosis, effective treatment, and follow-up.[111] Based on these recommendations, the Centers for Medicare and Medicaid Services recently determined to cover annual screening for depression for Medicare beneficiaries in primary care settings with staff-assisted depression care supports.

TREATMENT STRATEGIES

In managing DM, clinicians use several clinical data to establish baseline and treatment goals (eg, fasting serum glucose level and HgA1C). The same stepped, measurement-based treatment principles can be applied to treating depression: establishing a baseline; setting clinical and functional goals for depression; and assessing the patient's progress accordingly. **Fig. 2** illustrates one of the widely used clinical guidelines for depression treatment.

Various treatment options are available for late-life depression: antidepressant medications, psychotherapy, or a combination. Other options include exercise programs or other lifestyle-modifying interventions and electroconvulsive therapy (ECT).

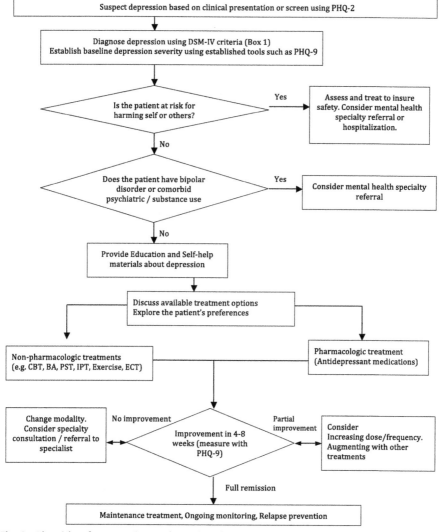

Fig. 2. Algorithm for screening and treating depression in primary care setting. BA, Behavioral Activation and Pleasant Activity Scheduling; CBT, cognitive behavioral therapy; IPT, interpersonal therapy; PST, problem-solving treatment.

Several meta-analyses showed that combination therapy is more efficacious than monotherapeutic approaches in treating and in preventing relapse.[112–115] In a recent meta-analysis of 14 randomized controlled trials (RCTs) of intervention for depression among patients with diabetes, all treatments have been shown to be effective in the reduction of depressive symptoms (g = −0.51, 95% CI: −0.63 to −0.39).[116] The pooled effect size was large in psychotherapeutic interventions combined with diabetes self-management education (g = −0.58, 95% CI −0.77 to −0.39); pharmacologic treatment showed moderate pooled effect size (g = −0.47; 95% CI −0.67 to −0.27).[116] Unlike major depression, subsyndromal depressive conditions have a relatively small evidence base regarding treatments; existing data suggest that available therapies have modest effect sizes when compared with usual care or placebo.[16,117,118]

Targeting interventions for patients with minor and subsyndromal depression may prove useful as both primary and secondary prevention strategies and clinicians should watch such patients carefully because of the high risk of worsening depression, especially if patients have experienced prior episodes of major depression. Psychosocial treatments may be more helpful than medications for older adults with less severe forms of depression.[119]

Treatment Delivery Model for Comorbid Depression and Diabetes Mellitus

To date, more than 40 RCTs have established a robust evidence base for an approach called collaborative care models (also called integrated care models).[120–123] Recently, several trials of collaborative care model have documented the effectiveness of treating comorbid depression and DM[123,124] (eg, PATHWAY[124]) and comorbid depression, and DM and/or coronary heart disease (TEAMcare[125]). In such programs, a depression care manager (usually a nurse or clinical social worker) supports medication management prescribed by primary care physicians (PCPs) through patient education, close and proactive follow-up, and brief, evidence-based psychosocial treatments, such as behavioral activation or problem-solving treatment in primary care. The care manager may also facilitate referrals to additional services as needed. A psychiatric consultant regularly (usually weekly) reviews all patients in the care manager's caseload who are not improving as expected and provides focused treatment recommendations to the patient's PCP.[120,126–128]

Tools for Assessing and Tracking Depression

Several tools for assessing depression severity are available and can be easily administered by office staff or physicians during a clinic care visit. The most frequently used tool is the 9-item Patient Health Questionnaire (PHQ-9),[129] which systematically explores the 9 DSM-IV[130] symptoms of major depression. A score of 10 or greater on the PHQ-9 indicates an elevated level of depressive symptoms and increased risk of clinically significant depression. PHQ-9 has good sensitivity and specificity (both about 88%) for detecting depressive disorders.[129,131]

Pharmacologic Management

Approximately 80% of the antidepressantd prescribed in the United States is prescribed in primary care settings. More than 20 antidepressant medications have been approved by the US Food and Drug Administration for the treatment of depression in older adults. Newer generations of antidepressants, such as selective serotonin-reuptake inhibitors and serotonin-norepinephrine reuptake inhibitors, have a more tolerable side-effect profile compared with tricyclic antidepressants.[132,133] Comparing second-generation antidepressants, studies found no evidence that specific medications are more effective than others.[134] Thus, physicians may discuss the choice of

Table 2
Commonly used antidepressant for late-life depression

Medication	Starting Dose	Common Therapeutic Doses	Half-life (h)	Common Side Effects	Comments
Selective serotonin-reuptake inhibitors					
Fluoxetine	5 mg	10–40 mg once daily	70–80	Nausea, dyspepsia, anorexia, tremors, anxiety, insomnia, sexual dysfunction, jitteriness, hyponatremia	Risk of serotonin syndrome if combined with certain drugs
					Very long acting
Sertraline	12.5 mg	50–200 mg once daily	25–30	Loose stools, diarrhea	
Citalopram	10 mg	20–40 mg once daily	40–50		
Escitalopram	2.5 mg	10–30 mg once daily	40–50		
Paroxetine	10 mg	20–50 mg once daily	10–20	Dry mouth, drowsiness, fatigue, weight gain	More anticholinergic side effects. High risk of discontinuation syndrome if drug stopped abruptly
Serotonin-norepinephrine reuptake inhibitors					
				Nausea, drowsiness, fatigue, weight gain, hyponatremia, diastolic hypertension at higher doses	Risk of serotonin syndrome if combined with certain drugs. High risk of discontinuation syndrome if medication stopped abruptly
Venlafaxine XR	37.5 mg	75–225 g once daily	5–9		
Duloxetine	20 mg	20–60 mg once daily	8–17		
Other newer antidepressants					
Mirtazapine	15 mg	15–45 mg at bedtime	20–40	Sedation, increased appetite/weight gain	No sexual side effects
Bupropion SR	100 mg	100–150 mg twice daily	15		No sexual side effects. Contraindicated in patients with seizures. Not recommended for patients with comorbid anxiety
Tricyclic antidepressants				Sedation, weight gain, dry mouth, urinary retention, constipation, blurry vision, orthostatic hypotension, impairment of cardiac conduction	High risk of overdose: 10 d of typical daily dose may result in a fatal cardiac arrhythmia. Get baseline ECG and follow-up ECG at steady state or if new cardiac symptoms occur
Nortriptyline	10 mg	50–125 mg every night	18–56	Fatigue	Therapeutic blood levels range from 50 to 150 ng/mL
Desipramine	25 mg	100–200 mg once daily	12–28	Insomnia, agitation	

medication with patients and their family. Because of the changes in pharmacokinetics (eg, decreased renal or hepatic clearance), older adults may require lower doses of medications than their younger counterparts. Furthermore, considering high rates of multimorbidity and polypharmacy among older adults, drug-drug interactions are a particular concern in this population. On the other hand, medication doses should be titrated upwards to full adult doses in patients who experience partial responses without substantial side effects. **Table 2** summarizes common antidepressant medications.

Psychological Management

Older adults patients with depression tend to prefer psychotherapy over medications.[135] Several psychotherapeutic modalities are effective for late-life depression[136–138]: cognitive behavioral therapy,[119,139] interpersonal therapy,[140] problem-solving treatment,[141] and Behavioral Activation and Pleasant Activity Scheduling.[142–144] A recent meta-analysis of 44 studies comparing psychotherapies and control conditions[138] concluded that the overall effect size of psychotherapy over control group was g = 0.64 (95% CI: 0.47–0.80). Although such treatments can be effectively provided to older adults in primary care,[145,146] they are not widely available in most primary care settings today and

Table 3
Efficacious nonpharmacologic treatments for late-life depression

Treatment Type	Studies	Level of Evidence	Comments
Cognitive behavioral therapy (CBT)	Gould et al,[157] 2012	Meta-analysis of RCTs	CBT significantly more efficacious at reducing depressive symptoms Combination with pharmacotherapy more efficacious than CBT alone
	Cuijpers et al,[138] 2014	Meta-analysis of RCTs	Older adults populations studies
Behavior activation (BA)	Cuijpers et al,[142] 2007	Meta-analysis of RCTs	Mixed population studies Effect is weaker in older adults
	Ekers et al,[158] 2014	Meta-analysis of RCTs	Mixed population studies
	Samad et al,[159] 2011	Meta-analysis of RCTs	Older adults populations studies
Problem-solving therapy	Bell et al,[141] 2009	Meta-analysis of RCTs	Mixed population studies
Interpersonal psychotherapy	Beekman et al,[160] 2006	Pragmatic RCT	Older adults populations studies
Reminiscence (life review)	Bohlmeijer et al,[161] 2003	Meta-analysis of RCTs	Older adults populations studies
	Pinquart & Forstmeier,[162] 2012	Meta-analysis of RCTs	Efficacious for broad range of outcomes, and therapeutic as well as preventive effects are similar to those observed in other frequently used interventions

clinicians are encouraged to develop relationships with mental health specialists who can offer such treatments or to train a staff member in the clinic to provide evidence-based brief psychotherapies. **Table 3** summarizes brief and evidence-based psycho-therapeutic approaches that can be easily administered in the primary care context and by nurses, social workers, or other licensed psychotherapists.

Electroconvulsive Treatment

ECT is an important and viable treatment option for severely depressed older adults. ECT should be strongly considered for patients who have severe, persistent depression that does not respond to several trials of antidepressant medications or psychotherapy and/or puts patient at high risk of harm (eg, severe weight loss, malnutrition, refusal of food, suicidal ideation). Poor tolerance or limited response to medications and a history of successful treatment with ECT are also indications for ECT. Rates of ECT use in depressed adults vary substantially.[147–149] Older adults are more likely to receive ECT than younger adults; African Americans are less likely to receive ECT than whites, and individuals with poor health insurance or living in rural areas are also less likely to receive ECT.[147]

SUMMARY

DM and depression are frequently comorbid in older adult patients. Considering the negative synergistic effects on the range of health outcomes resulted by comorbid depression and DM, prevention and early treatment of comorbid depression are a critical component of successful health management in older adult patients with DM.

REFERENCES

1. Centers for Disease Control Prevention. National diabetes fact sheet: national estimates and general information on diabetes and prediabetes in the United States. Atlanta (GA): US Department of Health and Human Services; Centers for Disease Control and Prevention; 2011. p. 201.
2. Park M, Katon WJ, Wolf FM. Depression and risk of mortality in individuals with diabetes: a meta-analysis and systematic review. Gen Hosp Psychiatry 2013; 35(3):217–25.
3. Cuijpers P, Beekman AT, Reynolds CF 3rd. Preventing depression: a global priority. JAMA 2012;307(10):1033–4.
4. Palinkas L, Barrett-Connor E, Wingard D. Type 2 diabetes and depressive symptoms in older adults: a population-based study. Diabet Med 1991;8(6): 532–9.
5. Kramer MK, Kriska AM, Venditti EM, et al. Translating the Diabetes Prevention Program: a comprehensive model for prevention training and program delivery. Am J Prev Med 2009;37(6):505–11.
6. Murray CJ, Lopez AD. Measuring the global burden of disease. N Engl J Med 2013;369(5):448–57.
7. Park M, Unützer J. Public Health Burden of Late-Life Mood Disorders. In: Levretsky H, Sajatovic M, Reynolds C, editors. Late-life Mood Disorders. New York: Oxford University Press; 2013. p. 42–60.
8. Anderson RJ, Freedland KE, Clouse RE, et al. The prevalence of comorbid depression in adults with diabetes: a meta-analysis. Diabetes Care 2001; 24(6):1069–78.
9. Ludman EJ, Katon W, Russo J, et al. Depression and diabetes symptom burden. Gen Hosp Psychiatry 2004;26(6):430–6.

10. Gonzalez JS, Peyrot M, McCarl LA, et al. Depression and diabetes treatment nonadherence: a meta-analysis. Diabetes Care 2008;31(12):2398–403.
11. Egede LE, Zheng D, Simpson K. Comorbid depression is associated with increased health care use and expenditures in individuals with diabetes. Diabetes Care 2002;25(3):464–70.
12. de Groot M, Anderson R, Freedland KE, et al. Association of depression and diabetes complications: a meta-analysis. Psychosom Med 2001;63(4):619–30.
13. Katon W, Lyles CR, Parker MM, et al. Association of depression with increased risk of dementia in patients with type 2 diabetes: the Diabetes and Aging Study. Arch Gen Psychiatry 2012;69(4):410–7.
14. Blazer DG. Psychiatry and the oldest old. Am J Psychiatry 2000;157(12): 1915–24.
15. Evans DL, Charney DS, Lewis L, et al. Mood disorders in the medically ill: scientific review and recommendations. Biol Psychiatry 2005;58(3):175–89.
16. Unutzer J. Diagnosis and treatment of older adults with depression in primary care. Biol Psychiatry 2002;52(3):285–92.
17. Lyness JM, Kim J, Tang W, et al. The clinical significance of subsyndromal depression in older primary care patients. Am J Geriatr Psychiatry 2007;15(3): 214–23, 210.1097/1001.JGP.0000235763.0000250230.0000235783.
18. Meeks TW, Vahia IV, Lavretsky H, et al. A tune in "a minor" can "b major": a review of epidemiology, illness course, and public health implications of subthreshold depression in older adults. J Affect Disord 2011;129(1–3):126–42.
19. Judd LL, Akiskal HS. The clinical and public health relevance of current research on subthreshold depressive symptoms to elderly patients. Am J Geriatr Psychiatry 2002;10(3):233–8.
20. Lavretsky H, Kumar A. Clinically significant non-major depression: old concepts, new insights. Am J Geriatr Psychiatry 2002;10(3):239–55.
21. Lyness J, King D, Cox C, et al. The importance of subsyndromal depression in older primary care patients: prevalence and associated functional disability. J Am Geriatr Soc 1999;47(6):647–52.
22. Remick RA. Diagnosis and management of depression in primary care: a clinical update and review. CMAJ 2002;167(11):1253–60.
23. Lyness JM, Yu Q, Tang W, et al. Risks for depression onset in primary care elderly patients: potential targets for preventive interventions. Am J Psychiatry 2009;166(12):1375–83.
24. Grabovich A, Lu N, Tang W, et al. Outcomes of subsyndromal depression in older primary care patients. Am J Geriatr Psychiatry 2010;18(3):227–35.
25. Unutzer J. Clinical practice. Late-life depression. N Engl J Med 2007;357(22): 2269–76.
26. Klein DN, Shankman SA, Rose S. Ten-year prospective follow-up study of the naturalistic course of dysthymic disorder and double depression. Am J Psychiatry 2006;163(5):872–80.
27. Mueller TI, Leon AC, Keller MB, et al. Recurrence after recovery from major depressive disorder during 15 years of observational follow-up. Am J Psychiatry 1999;156(7):1000–6.
28. Licht-Strunk E, van der Windt DA, van Marwijk HW, et al. The prognosis of depression in older patients in general practice and the community. A systematic review. Fam Pract 2007;24(2):168–80.
29. Cole MG, Bellavance F, Mansour A. Prognosis of depression in elderly community and primary care populations: a systematic review and meta-analysis. Am J Psychiatry 1999;156(8):1182–9.

30. Iosifescu DV, Nierenberg AA, Alpert JE, et al. Comorbid medical illness and relapse of major depressive disorder in the continuation phase of treatment. Psychosomatics 2004;45(5):419–25.
31. Fisher L, Skaff MM, Mullan JT, et al. Clinical depression versus distress among patients with type 2 diabetes not just a question of semantics. Diabetes Care 2007;30(3):542–8.
32. Drayer RA, Mulsant BH, Lenze EJ, et al. Somatic symptoms of depression in elderly patients with medical comorbidities. Int J Geriatr Psychiatry 2005; 20(10):973–82.
33. Kirmayer LJ, Young A. Culture and somatization: clinical, epidemiological, and ethnographic perspectives. Psychosom Med 1998;60(4):420–30.
34. Sadovnick AD, Remick RA, Lam R, et al. Mood disorder service genetic database: morbidity risks for mood disorders in 3,942 first-degree relatives of 671 index cases with single depression, recurrent depression, bipolar I, or bipolar II. Am J Med Genet 1994;54(2):132–40.
35. Stroebe M, Schut H, Stroebe W. Health outcomes of bereavement. Lancet 2007; 370(9603):1960–73.
36. Pinquart M, Sorensen S. Influences of socioeconomic status, social network, and competence on subjective well-being in later life: a meta-analysis. Psychol Aging 2000;15(2):187–224.
37. Park M, Unützer J, Grembowski D. Ethnic and gender variations in the associations between family cohesion, family conflict, and depression in older Asian and Latino adults. J Immigr Minor Health 2013. [Epub ahead of print].
38. Park M, Unutzer J. Hundred forty eight more days with depression: the association between marital conflict and depression-free days. Int J Geriatr Psychiatry 2014. [Epub ahead of print].
39. Thompson A, Fan MY, Unutzer J, et al. One extra month of depression: the effects of caregiving on depression outcomes in the IMPACT trial. Int J Geriatr Psychiatry 2008;23(5):511–6.
40. Abe-Kim J, Takeuchi DT, Hong S, et al. Use of mental health-related services among immigrant and US-born Asian Americans: results from the National Latino and Asian American study. Am J Public Health 2007;97(1):91–8.
41. Abe-Kim JS, Takeuchi DT. Cultural competence and quality of care: issues for mental health service delivery in managed care. Clin Psychol Sci Pract 1996; 3(4):273–95.
42. Aber JL, Bennett NG, Conley DC, et al. The effects of poverty on child health and development. Annu Rev Public Health 1997;18:463–83.
43. Abueg FR, Chun KM. Traumatization stress among Asians and Asian Americans. In: Marsella AJ, Friedman MJ, Gerrity E, et al, editors. Ethnocultural aspects of posttraumatic stress disorder: issues, research, and clinical applications. Washington, DC: American Psychological Association; 1996. p. 285–99.
44. Ackerman DL, Unutzer J, Greenland S, et al. Inpatient treatment of depression and associated hospital charges. Pharmacoepidemiol Drug Saf 2002;11(3): 219–27.
45. Adler N, Boyce W, Chesney M, et al. Socioeconomic inequalities in health: no easy solution. JAMA 1993;269:3140.
46. Adler NE, Newman K. Socioeconomic disparities in health: pathways and policies. Health Aff (Millwood) 2002;21(2):60–76.
47. Park M. The variations in associations between family contexts and late-life depression outcomes [thesis]. Seattle WA: Health Services, University of Washington; 2013.

48. Martire LM, Schulz R. Involving family in psychosocial interventions for chronic illness. Curr Dir Psychol Sci 2007;16(2):90–4.
49. Lee MS, Crittenden KS, Yu E. Social support and depression among elderly Korean immigrants in the United States. Int J Aging Hum Dev 1996;42(4): 313–27.
50. George LK, Blazer DG, Hughes DC, et al. Social support and the outcome of major depression. Br J Psychiatry 1989;154(4):478–85.
51. Smith F, Francis SA, Gray N, et al. A multi-centre survey among informal carers who manage medication for older care recipients: problems experienced and development of services. Health Soc Care Community 2003;11(2):138–45.
52. Voils CI, Steffens DC, Flint EP, et al. Social support and locus of control as predictors of adherence to antidepressant medication in an elderly population. Am J Geriatr Psychiatry 2005;13(2):157–65.
53. National Healthcare Disparities Report. Rockville (MD): Agency for Healthcare Research and Quality; 2004.
54. National Healthcare Disparities Report. Rockville (MD): Agency for Healthcare Research and Quality; 2007.
55. Kawachi I, Berkman L. Social ties and mental health. J Urban Health 2001;78(3): 458–67.
56. Hong SI, Hasche L, Bowland S. Structural relationships between social activities and longitudinal trajectories of depression among older adults. Gerontologist 2009;49(1):1–11.
57. Unutzer J, Katon W, Sullivan M, et al. Treating depressed older adults in primary care: narrowing the gap between efficacy and effectiveness. Milbank Q 1999; 77(2):225–56, 174.
58. Centers for Disease Control and Prevention, National Association of Chronic Disease Directors. The state of mental health and aging in America issue brief 2: addressing depression in older adults: selected evidence-based programs. In: National Association of chronic disease directors, editor. Atlanta (GA): 2009.
59. Kessler RC, Berglund P, Demler O, et al. Lifetime prevalence and age-of-onset distributions of DSM-IV disorders in the National Comorbidity Survey Replication. Arch Gen Psychiatry 2005;62(6):593–602.
60. Mojtabai R, Olfson M. Major depression in community-dwelling middle-aged and older adults: prevalence and 2- and 4-year follow-up symptoms. Psychol Med 2004;34(04):623–34.
61. Byers AL, Yaffe K, Covinsky KE, et al. High occurrence of mood and anxiety disorders among older adults: the National Comorbidity Survey Replication. Arch Gen Psychiatry 2010;67(5):489–96.
62. Blazer DG. Depression in late life: review and commentary. Focus 2009;7(1): 118–36.
63. Teresi J, Abrams R, Holmes D, et al. Prevalence of depression and depression recognition in nursing homes. Soc Psychiatry Psychiatr Epidemiol 2001;36(12): 613–20.
64. Hoover DR, Siegel M, Lucas J, et al. Depression in the first year of stay for elderly long-term nursing home residents in the U.S.A. Int Psychogeriatr 2010; 22:1161–71.
65. Lyness JM, Caine ED, King DA, et al. Psychiatric disorders in older primary care patients. J Gen Intern Med 1999;14(4):249–54.
66. Kuo BCH, Chong V, Joseph J. Depression and its psychosocial correlates among older Asian immigrants in North America. J Aging Health 2008;20(6): 615–52.

67. Simpson S, Krishnan L, Kunik M, et al. Racial disparities in diagnosis and treatment of depression: a literature review. Psychiatr Q 2007;78(1):3–14.
68. Black SA, Markides KS, Ray LA. Depression predicts increased incidence of adverse health outcomes in older Mexican Americans with type 2 diabetes. Diabetes Care 2003;26(10):2822–8.
69. Steffens DC, Fisher GG, Langa KM, et al. Prevalence of depression among older Americans: the Aging, Demographics and Memory Study. Int Psychogeriatr 2009;21(5):879–88.
70. Strothers HS, Rust G, Minor P, et al. Disparities in antidepressant treatment in Medicaid elderly diagnosed with depression. J Am Geriatr Soc 2005;53(3):456–61.
71. Crystal S, Sambamoorthi U, Walkup JT, et al. Diagnosis and treatment of depression in the elderly Medicare population: predictors, disparities, and trends. J Am Geriatr Soc 2003;51(12):1718–28.
72. Kleinman A. Patients and healers in the context of culture: an exploration of the borderland between anthropology, medicine, and psychiatry. Berkeley, Los Angeles (CA): University of California Press; 1981.
73. Kleinman A. Culture and depression. N Engl J Med 2004;351(10):951–3.
74. Pang KY. Symptom expression and somatization among elderly Korean immigrants. J Clin Geropsychol 2000;6(3):199–212.
75. Jackson JL, Kroenke K. Difficult patient encounters in the ambulatory clinic: clinical predictors and outcomes. Arch Intern Med 1999;159(10):1069–75.
76. Cooper LA, Gonzales JJ, Gallo JJ, et al. The acceptability of treatment for depression among African-American, Hispanic, and white primary care patients. Med Care 2003;41(4):479–89.
77. Givens JL, Houston TK, Van Voorhees BW, et al. Ethnicity and preferences for depression treatment. Gen Hosp Psychiatry 2007;29(3):182–91.
78. Alegria M, Chatterji P, Wells K, et al. Disparity in depression treatment among racial and ethnic minority populations in the United States. Psychiatr Serv 2008;59(11):1264–72.
79. Kessler RC, Birnbaum HG, Shahly V, et al. Age differences in the prevalence and co-morbidity of DSM-IV major depressive episodes: results from the WHO World Mental Health Survey Initiative. Depress Anxiety 2010;27(4):351–64.
80. Chen L, Magliano DJ, Zimmet PZ. The worldwide epidemiology of type 2 diabetes mellitus–present and future perspectives. Nat Rev Endocrinol 2012;8(4):228–36.
81. Wild S, Roglic G, Green A, et al. Global prevalence of diabetes: estimates for the year 2000 and projections for 2030. Diabetes Care 2004;27(5):1047–53.
82. Ali S, Stone MA, Peters JL, et al. The prevalence of co-morbid depression in adults with Type 2 diabetes: a systematic review and meta-analysis. Diabet Med 2006;23(11):1165–73.
83. Li C, Ford E, Strine T, et al. Prevalence of depression among U.S. adults with diabetes: findings from the 2006 behavioral risk factor surveillance system. Diabetes Care 2008;31:105.
84. Hofmann M, Köhler B, Leichsenring F, et al. Depression as a risk factor for mortality in individuals with diabetes: a meta-analysis of prospective studies. PLoS One 2013;8(11):e79809.
85. van Dooren FE, Nefs G, Schram MT, et al. Depression and risk of mortality in people with diabetes mellitus: a systematic review and meta-analysis. PLoS One 2013;8(3):e57058.
86. Bogner HR, Morales KH, Post EP, et al. Diabetes, depression, and death: a randomized controlled trial of a depression treatment program for older adults based in primary care (PROSPECT). Diabetes Care 2007;30(12):3005–10.

87. Gallo JJ, Morales KH, Bogner HR, et al. Long term effect of depression care management on mortality in older adults: follow-up of cluster randomized clinical trial in primary care. BMJ 2013;346:f2570.

88. Katon WJ. Clinical and health services relationships between major depression, depressive symptoms, and general medical illness. Biol Psychiatry 2003;54(3): 216–26.

89. Golden S, Lazo M, Carnethon M, et al. Examining a bidirectional association between depressive symptoms and diabetes. JAMA 2008;299:2751.

90. Stuart MJ, Baune BT. Depression and type 2 diabetes: inflammatory mechanisms of a psychoneuroendocrine co-morbidity. Neurosci Biobehav Rev 2012; 36(1):658–76.

91. Silva N, Atlantis E, Ismail K. A review of the association between depression and insulin resistance: pitfalls of secondary analyses or a promising new approach to prevention of type 2 diabetes? Curr Psychiatry Rep 2012;14(1):8–14.

92. Feinkohl I, Aung PP, Keller M, et al. Severe hypoglycemia and cognitive decline in older people with type 2 diabetes: the Edinburgh Type 2 Diabetes Study. Diabetes care 2014;37(2):507–15.

93. Ciechanowski PS, Katon WJ, Russo JE, et al. The relationship of depressive symptoms to symptom reporting, self-care and glucose control in diabetes. Gen Hosp Psychiatry 2003;25(4):246–52.

94. Ciechanowski PS, Katon WJ, Russo JE. Depression and diabetes: impact of depressive symptoms on adherence, function, and costs. Arch Intern Med 2000;160(21):3278–85.

95. McDermott LM, Ebmeier KP. A meta-analysis of depression severity and cognitive function. J Affect Disord 2009;119(1–3):1–8.

96. Byers AL, Yaffe K. Depression and risk of developing dementia. Nat Rev Neurol 2011;7(6):323–31.

97. Rapp MA, Schnaider-Beeri M, Wysocki M, et al. Cognitive decline in patients with dementia as a function of depression. Am J Geriatr Psychiatry 2011; 19(4):357–63.

98. Stetler C, Miller GE. Depression and hypothalamic-pituitary-adrenal activation: a quantitative summary of four decades of research. Psychosom Med 2011;73(2): 114–26.

99. Lok A, Mocking RJ, Ruhe HG, et al. Longitudinal hypothalamic-pituitary-adrenal axis trait and state effects in recurrent depression. Psychoneuroendocrinology 2012;37(7):892–902.

100. Vanhanen M, Koivisto K, Moilanen L, et al. Association of metabolic syndrome with Alzheimer disease a population-based study. Neurology 2006;67(5):843–7.

101. Craft S. The role of metabolic disorders in Alzheimer disease and vascular dementia: two roads converged. Arch Neurol 2009;66(3):300–5.

102. Notarianni E. Hypercortisolemia and glucocorticoid receptor-signaling insufficiency in Alzheimer's disease initiation and development. Curr Alzheimer Res 2013;10(7):714–31.

103. Cole J, Costafreda SG, McGuffin P, et al. Hippocampal atrophy in first episode depression: a meta-analysis of magnetic resonance imaging studies. J Affect Disord 2011;134(1–3):483–7.

104. Taylor WD, McQuoid DR, Payne ME, et al. Hippocampus atrophy and the longitudinal course of late-life depression. Am J Geriatr Psychiatry 2013. [Epub ahead of print].

105. Mezuk B, Eaton WW, Albrecht S, et al. Depression and type 2 diabetes over the lifespan: a meta-analysis. Diabetes Care 2008;31(12):2383–90.

106. Demakakos P, Pierce MB, Hardy R. Depressive symptoms and risk of type 2 diabetes in a national sample of middle-aged and older adults. Diabetes Care 2010;33(4):792–7.
107. Carnethon MR, Kinder LS, Fair JM, et al. Symptoms of depression as a risk factor for incident diabetes: findings from the National Health and Nutrition Examination Epidemiologic Follow-up Study, 1971–1992. Am J Epidemiol 2003; 158(5):416–23.
108. Eaton W, Pratt L, Armenian H, et al. Depression and risk for onset of type II diabetes. A prospective population-based study. Diabetes Care 1996;19:1097–102.
109. Nouwen A, Winkley K, Twisk J, et al. Type 2 diabetes mellitus as a risk factor for the onset of depression: a systematic review and meta-analysis. Diabetologia 2010;53(12):2480–6.
110. Reynolds CF, Thomas SB, Morse JQ, et al. Early intervention to preempt major depression among older black and white adults. Psychiatr Serv 2014;65(6): 765–73.
111. U.S. Preventive Services Task Force. Screening for Depression: Recommendations and Rationale. 2002. Available at: http://www.uspreventiveservicestaskforce.org/3rduspstf/depression/depressrr.htm. Accessed October 30, 2011.
112. Cuijpers P, van Straten A, Hollon SD, et al. The contribution of active medication to combined treatments of psychotherapy and pharmacotherapy for adult depression: a meta-analysis. Acta Psychiatr Scand 2010;121(6):415–23.
113. Kohler S, Hoffmann S, Unger T, et al. Effectiveness of cognitive-behavioural therapy plus pharmacotherapy in inpatient treatment of depressive disorders. Clin Psychol Psychother 2013;20(2):97–106.
114. Rocha FL, Fuzikawa C, Riera R, et al. Combination of antidepressants in the treatment of major depressive disorder: a systematic review and meta-analysis. J Clin Psychopharmacol 2012;32(2):278–81.
115. Reynolds CF, Frank E, Perel JM, et al. Nortriptyline and interpersonal psychotherapy as maintenance therapies for recurrent major depression. JAMA 1999;281(1):39–45.
116. van der Feltz-Cornelis CM, Nuyen J, Stoop C, et al. Effect of interventions for major depressive disorder and significant depressive symptoms in patients with diabetes mellitus: a systematic review and meta-analysis. Gen Hosp Psychiatry 2010;32(4):380–95.
117. Bruce ML, Ten Have TR, Reynolds CF III, et al. Reducing suicidal ideation and depressive symptoms in depressed older primary care patients: a randomized controlled trial. JAMA 2004;291(9):1081–91.
118. Oxman TE, Sengupta A. Treatment of minor depression. Am J Geriatr Psychiatry 2002;10(3):256–64.
119. Pinquart M, Duberstein PR, Lyness JM. Treatments for later-life depressive conditions: a meta-analytic comparison of pharmacotherapy and psychotherapy. Am J Psychiatry 2006;163(9):1493–501.
120. Gilbody S, Bower P, Fletcher J, et al. Collaborative care for depression: a cumulative meta-analysis and review of longer-term outcomes. Arch Intern Med 2006; 166:2314–21.
121. Simon G. Collaborative care for depression. BMJ 2006;332(7536):249–50.
122. Simon G. Collaborative care for mood disorders. Curr Opin Psychiatry 2009; 22(1):37–41.
123. Bogner HR, Morales KH, de Vries HF, et al. Integrated management of type 2 diabetes mellitus and depression treatment to improve medication adherence: a randomized controlled trial. Ann Fam Med 2012;10(1):15–22.

124. Katon W, Von Korff M, Lin EH, et al. The Pathways Study: a randomized trial of collaborative care in patients with diabetes and depression. Arch Gen Psychiatry 2004;61(10):1042–9.
125. Katon W, Lin EH, Von Korff M, et al. Integrating depression and chronic disease care among patients with diabetes and/or coronary heart disease: the design of the TEAMcare study. Contemp Clin Trials 2010;31(4):312–22.
126. Katon W, Unutzer J. Collaborative care models for depression: time to move from evidence to practice. Arch Intern Med 2006;166(21):2304–6.
127. Katon W, Unutzer J, Wells K, et al. Collaborative depression care: history, evolution and ways to enhance dissemination and sustainability. Gen Hosp Psychiatry 2010;32(5):456–64.
128. Katon W, Von Korff M, Lin E, et al. Rethinking practitioner roles in chronic illness: the specialist, primary care physician, and the practice nurse. Gen Hosp Psychiatry 2001;23(3):138–44.
129. Kroenke K, Spitzer RL, Williams JBW, et al. The patient health questionnaire somatic, anxiety, and depressive symptom scales: a systematic review. Gen Hosp Psychiatry 2010;32(4):345–59.
130. American Psychiatric Association. Diagnostic and statistical manual of mental disorders: DSM-IV-TR. 4th edition. Washington, DC: American Psychiatric Association; 2000.
131. Kroenke K, Spitzer RL, Williams JB. The patient health questionnaire-2: validity of a two-item depression screener. Med Care 2003;41(11):1284–92.
132. Kok RM, Heeren TJ, Nolen WA. Continuing treatment of depression in the elderly: a systematic review and meta-analysis of double-blinded randomized controlled trials with antidepressants. Am J Geriatr Psychiatry 2011;19(3): 249–55, 210.1097/JGP.1090b1013e3181ec8085.
133. Nelson JC, Delucchi K, Schneider L. Efficacy of second generation antidepressants in late-life depression: a meta-analysis of the evidence. Am J Geriatr Psychiatry 2008;16(7):558–67.
134. Gartlehner G, Gaynes BN, Hansen RA, et al. Comparative benefits and harms of second-generation antidepressants: background paper for the American College of Physicians. Ann Intern Med 2008;149(10):734–50.
135. Gum AM, Arean PA, Hunkeler E, et al. Depression treatment preferences in older primary care patients. Gerontologist 2006;46(1):14–22.
136. Cuijpers P, van Straten A, Smit F. Psychological treatment of late-life depression: a meta-analysis of randomized controlled trials. Int J Geriatr Psychiatry 2006; 21(12):1139–49.
137. Pinquart M, Duberstein PR, Lyness JM. Effects of psychotherapy and other behavioral interventions on clinically depressed older adults: a meta-analysis. Aging Ment Health 2007;11(6):645–57.
138. Cuijpers P, Karyotaki E, Pot AM, et al. Managing depression in older age: psychological interventions. Maturitas 2014;79(2):160–9.
139. Wilson KC, Mottram PG, Vassilas CA. Psychotherapeutic treatments for older depressed people. Cochrane Database Syst Rev 2008;(1):CD004853.
140. de Mello MF, de Jesus Mari J, Bacaltchuk J, et al. A systematic review of research findings on the efficacy of interpersonal therapy for depressive disorders. Eur Arch Psychiatry Clin Neurosci 2005;255(2):75–82.
141. Bell AC, D'Zurilla TJ. Problem-solving therapy for depression: a meta-analysis. Clin Psychol Rev 2009;29(4):348–53.
142. Cuijpers P, van Straten A, Warmerdam L. Behavioral activation treatments of depression: a meta-analysis. Clin Psychol Rev 2007;27(3):318–26.

143. Mazzucchelli T, Kane R, Rees C. Behavioral activation treatments for depression in adults: a meta-analysis and review. Clin Psychol Sci Pract 2009;16(4):383–411.

144. Ekers D, Richards D, Gilbody S. A meta-analysis of randomized trials of behavioural treatment of depression. Psychol Med 2008;38(5):611–23.

145. Arean P, Hegel M, Vannoy S, et al. Effectiveness of problem-solving therapy for older, primary care patients with depression: results from the IMPACT project. Gerontologist 2008;48(3):311–23.

146. Schulberg HC, Post EP, Raue PJ, et al. Treating late-life depression with interpersonal psychotherapy in the primary care sector. Int J Geriatr Psychiatry 2007; 22(2):106–14.

147. Olfson M, Marcus S, Sackeim HA, et al. Use of ECT for the inpatient treatment of recurrent major depression. Am J Psychiatry 1998;155:22–9.

148. Case BG, Bertollo DN, Laska EM, et al. Racial differences in the availability and use of electroconvulsive therapy for recurrent major depression. J Affect Disord 2012;136(3):359–65.

149. American Psychiatric Association. Diagnostic and statistical manual of mental disorders. 5th edition. Washington, DC: American Psychiatric Association; 2013.

150. Cole MG, Dendukuri N. Risk factors for depression among elderly community subjects: a systematic review and meta-analysis. Am J Psychiatry 2003; 160(6):1147–56.

151. Snowdon J. Is depression more prevalent in old age? Aust N Z J Psychiatry 2001;35(6):782–7.

152. Sonnenberg CM, Beekman AT, Deeg DJ, et al. Sex differences in late-life depression. Acta Psychiatr Scand 2000;101(4):286–92.

153. Zisook S, Shuchter SR. Depression through the first year after the death of a spouse. Am J Psychiatry 1991;148(10):1346–52.

154. Turvey CL, Carney C, Arndt S, et al. Conjugal loss and syndromal depression in a sample of elders aged 70 years or older. Am J Psychiatry 1999;156(10):1596–601.

155. Prince MJ, Harwood RH, Thomas A, et al. A prospective population-based cohort study of the effects of disablement and social milieu on the onset and maintenance of late-life depression. The Gospel Oak Project VII. Psychol Med 1998;28(2):337–50.

156. Cacioppo JT, Hughes ME, Waite LJ, et al. Loneliness as a specific risk factor for depressive symptoms: cross-sectional and longitudinal analyses. Psychol Aging 2006;21(1):140.

157. Gould RL, Coulson MC, Howard RJ. Cognitive behavioral therapy for depression in older people: a meta-analysis and meta-regression of randomized controlled trials. J Am Geriatr Soc 2012;60(10):1817–30.

158. Ekers D, Webster L, Van Straten A, et al. Behavioural activation for depression; an update of meta-analysis of effectiveness and sub group analysis. PLoS One 2014;9(6):e100100.

159. Samad Z, Brealey S, Gilbody S. The effectiveness of behavioural therapy for the treatment of depression in older adults: a meta-analysis. Int J Geriatr Psychiatry 2011;26(12):1211–20.

160. Beekman A, van Schaik A, van Marwijk H, et al. Interpersonal psychotherapy for elderly patients in primary care. Am J Geriatr Psychiatry 2006;14(9):777–86, 710.1097/1001.JGP.0000199341.0000125431.0000199344b.

161. Bohlmeijer E, Smit F, Cuijpers P. Effects of reminiscence and life review on late-life depression: a meta-analysis. Int J Geriatr Psychiatry 2003;18(12):1088–94.

162. Pinquart M, Forstmeier S. Effects of reminiscence interventions on psychosocial outcomes: a meta-analysis. Aging Ment Health 2012;16(5):541–58.

Obstructive Sleep Apnea and Type 2 Diabetes in Older Adults

Karoline Moon, MD, Naresh M. Punjabi, MD, PhD,
R. Nisha Aurora, MD*

KEYWORDS

- Obstructive sleep apnea • Central sleep apnea • Type 2 diabetes • Aging

KEY POINTS

- Obstructive sleep apnea (OSA) is associated with insulin resistance, glucose intolerance, and type 2 diabetes independent of confounding effects of age and obesity.
- Intermittent hypoxemia and sleep fragmentation in OSA trigger a wide repertoire of pathophysiological mechanisms that may be responsible for altering glucose homeostasis and increasing the risk for type 2 diabetes.
- Treatment of OSA is associated with improvements in daytime sleepiness and quality of life, and may also have a favorable impact on glycemic control and glucose metabolism.
- OSA and central sleep apnea are common in people with type 2 diabetes, particularly in the presence of autonomic neuropathy.
- Given the high prevalence of OSA and type 2 diabetes in older adults, presence of 1 condition should prompt the evaluation of the other.

INTRODUCTION

Given the global increase in prevalence of obesity, obstructive sleep apnea (OSA) is becoming an increasingly common and pervasive condition. It has been estimated that OSA affects 12 to 18 million people in the United States alone.[1] In addition to its well-established neurocognitive effects,[2] OSA has also been found to be an independent risk factor for hypertension,[3] cardiovascular disease,[4] and impaired glucose metabolism.[5] Cross-sectional studies of clinic and population-based samples suggest that up to 50% of patients with OSA have type 2 diabetes, and approximately 50% of patients with type 2 diabetes have moderate-to-severe OSA.[6,7] Although many of the

Dr N.M. Punjabi was supported by National Institutes of Health (HL075078). Dr. R. Nisha Aurora was supported by a grant from the American Sleep Medicine Foundation (116210) and the National Institutes of Health (HL118414).
Division of Pulmonary and Critical Care Medicine, Johns Hopkins University, School of Medicine, 5501 Hopkins Bayview Circle, Baltimore, MD 21224, USA
* Corresponding author.
E-mail address: raurora2@jhmi.edu

Clin Geriatr Med 31 (2015) 139–147
http://dx.doi.org/10.1016/j.cger.2014.08.023
0749-0690/15/$ – see front matter © 2015 Elsevier Inc. All rights reserved.

putative links between OSA and metabolic dysfunction are not well elucidated, it is likely that intermittent hypoxemia and sleep fragmentation, the 2 pathophysiological con-comitants of OSA, play a fundamental role in the development of insulin resistance, glucose intolerance, and type 2 diabetes. The central theme of this article is to provide a brief appraisal of the bidirectional nature of the association between OSA and type 2 diabetes given that both conditions are increasingly prevalent in older adults.

SLEEP APNEA: DISEASE DEFINITION AND RISK FACTORS

Sleep apnea is a group of chronic sleep-related breathing disorders that are charac-terized by the occurrence of disordered breathing events during sleep. These events are generally classified into 2 main types: obstructive and central. The classification of an event as obstructive or central depends whether, in the absence of airflow, there is ongoing respiratory effort. OSA, which is the most prevalent type of sleep apnea, is characterized by the predominance of recurrent obstructive events that result from partial or complete collapse of the upper airway during sleep. The ensuing cessation of airflow (apneas) or decrease in airflow (hypopneas) is associated with a decrease in oxyhemoglobin saturation and arousal from sleep. In OSA, apneas and hypopneas during sleep are associated with continued respiratory effort. In contrast, in central sleep apnea, the upper airway remains patent, and the apneas and hypopneas result during sleep from a decrease or lack of respiratory muscle effort. The apnea–hypo-pnea index (AHI), which is the number of apneas and hypopneas per hour of sleep, is used as the disease-defining metric for OSA and central sleep apnea. By conven-tion, the following thresholds are used to classify the severity of obstructive or central sleep apnea: normal (AHI <5 events/h), mild (AHI: 5.0–14.9 events/h), moderate (AHI: 15.0–29.9 events/h), or severe (AHI ≥30 events/h). Although OSA is by far the more common type, OSA and central sleep apnea can coexist in older adults. Data from several large population-based cohort studies have estimated the prevalence of OSA to vary in the range of 5.0% to 15.0%.[8] Even more gripping is the large number of people with OSA who remain undiagnosed, estimated to be 70% to 90% of those with OSA.[9] Risk factors for OSA include advancing age, male sex, family history, excess body fat, central obesity, large neck circumference, and craniofacial and upper airway abnormalities.[8] Other risk factors include family history, smoking, being post-menopausal, and nighttime alcohol use.

AGE AS A RISK FACTOR FOR SLEEP APNEA

Even in the absence of an underlying sleep disorder, older age is associated with impairments in sleep quality that can be related to either chronic medical or psychiatric conditions and/or changes in social situation.[10] The presence of a sleep disorder such as OSA can further impair sleep quality. Studies investigating prevalence of OSA have generally shown that it is an age-related condition, with older adults having a higher prevalence compared with younger adults.[11–15] Points estimates of OSA prevalence, however, vary across studies, in part, because of the heterogeneity in study samples including recruitment source (clinic vs community-based), distribution of factors such as sex and body weight, and the methods used to identify OSA. Undoubtedly, the highest prevalence of OSA is in older men, with estimates in the range of 13% to 44% for those between 59 and 99 years old.[11–15] Cross-sectional data on OSA prev-alence as a function of age suggest that prevalence increases in middle-aged adults, up to the sixth decade of life, with a subsequent plateau (**Fig. 1**).[16] Longitudinal data on older cohorts also indicate a plateau, or perhaps even a decline, in OSA prevalence in the elderly.[17,18] It is certainly possible that survivor bias could explain the lack of a

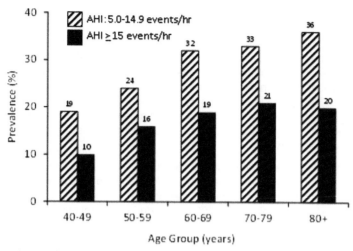

Fig. 1. Prevalence of obstructive sleep as a function of age.

monotonic increase in OSA prevalence with age, because the high prevalence of age-related comorbid conditions (eg, stroke, heart failure) may preclude participation of older adults in clinic and epidemiologic studies.

Risk factor profiles for OSA seem to vary as a function of increasing age. For example, body mass index (BMI) does not demonstrate the same strength of association in elderly adults as it does in young or middle-aged adults.[16,19–22] In fact, in the elderly, a declining trajectory of BMI has been associated with increasing OSA severity as assessed by the AHI.[22] A decrease in BMI, which may reflect loss of muscle mass, could be associated with decrease in functional activity of upper airway dilator muscles (eg, genioglossus) in the elderly.[23] Alterations in upper airway mechanics and anatomy (eg, increased pharyngeal fat pads or changes in bony structure) with aging can increase upper airway collapsibility and predispose to the occurrence of obstructive apneas and hypopneas during sleep.[23,24] Moreover, the higher prevalence of other chronic medical conditions such as congestive heart failure and stroke and the use of centrally acting medications (eg, opioids for chronic pain) can further escalate the risk for central sleep apnea and augment the untoward associated effects of intermittent hypoxemia and sleep disruption on health-related consequences. Thus, while BMI, central obesity, and sex have a substantial role in mediating OSA risk in younger and middle-aged adults, other factors have a greater influence on the development of obstructive or central sleep apnea in older adults. It is also important to recognize that the clinical manifestations and presentation of OSA can be distinct between older and younger or middle-aged adults. Reports of snoring, witnessed apneas, and other presenting symptoms for OSA are less common in older people than their younger counterparts.[16,25] Such differences underscore the importance of heightened vigilance in evaluating older patients if they report poor sleep quality or daytime sleepiness. In the sections that follow, the epidemiology of metabolic abnormalities is briefly reviewed, followed by an appraisal of the evidence on the bidirectional association between OSA and type 2 diabetes.

DISORDERS OF GLUCOSE OF METABOLISM: DEFINITION AND EPIDEMIOLOGY

Four distinct categories of diabetes mellitus have been proposed by the American Diabetes Association.[26] Type 1 diabetes, which accounts for 5% to 10% of all diabetes cases, develops as a result of pancreatic beta-cell destruction and associated impaired insulin secretion. In contrast, type 2 diabetes, which accounts for accounts 90% to 95% of all diabetes cases, is characterized by insulin resistance coupled with impairments in insulin secretion. Gestational diabetes is the third category of diabetes, which is diagnosed in the presence of any degree of glucose intolerance with onset of pregnancy and complicates about 4% of all pregnancies in the United States. Finally, the fourth category of diabetes includes genetic β-cell defects or defects in insulin action, pancreatic disease, endocrinopathies, drug-induced causes, infection, and genetic syndromes. The criteria for the diagnosis of diabetes require any of the following

1. Fasting blood glucose of at least 126 mg/dL
2. A random blood glucose of at least 200 mg/d and symptoms of hyperglycemia (ie, polyuria, polydipsia and unexplained weight loss)
3. 2-hour blood glucose of at least 200 mg/dL during an oral glucose tolerance test

In addition to the 4 categories of diabetes described previously, there are 2 clinically relevant prediabetic conditions, including impaired fasting glucose and impaired glucose tolerance. Impaired fasting glucose is defined as a fasting blood glucose level between 100 mg/dL and 126 mg/dL. Impaired glucose tolerance is defined as a 2-h blood glucose level between 140 mg/dL and 200 mg/dL during an oral glucose tolerance test.

Along with obesity, diabetes mellitus has also become a global epidemic, affecting approximately 7.7% of the world's population, with more than 90% of the cases being type 2 diabetics.[27] Prevalence estimates for type 2 diabetes range from 0.3% to17.9% in Africa, 1.2% to 14.6% in Asia, 0.7% to 11.6% in Europe, 4.6% to 40.0% in the Middle East, 6.7% to 28.2% in North America, and 2.0% to 17.4% in South America.[28] The development of type 2 diabetes is a complex, multistep process that is influenced by both genetic and environmental factors. Genetic susceptibility plays a significant role in the etiology of type 2 diabetes, as supported by studies of monozygotic twins, which show a concordance of nearly 100%.[29] Increased body fat, visceral adiposity, and sedentary life style are some other well-known risk factors for type 2 diabetes. Moreover, the increasing prevalence of diabetes over the past 20 years has been predominantly in people 65 years in age or older.[30] In fact, 40% of people in the United States and more than 50% of people worldwide with type 2 diabetes are over the age of 65 years. Furthermore, it is estimated that by the year 2050 there will be at least a 4.5-fold increase in the number of people over 65 years in age with type 2 diabetes.[30] The higher predisposition for developing type 2 diabetes with increasing age is caused by the age-related decrease in whole-body insulin sensitivity and insulin secretion from the pancreatic beta-cell. The decline in insulin insensitivity with age is attributable to muscle fat accumulation and a reduction in mitochondrial function in muscle.[31] Over the last 20 years, there has been increased recognition that OSA may also predispose to the development of type 2 diabetes, which, in turn, may over time worsen OSA severity and establish a potentially feed-forward loop as will be described.

OBSTRUCTIVE SLEEP APNEA AS A CAUSE OF METABOLIC DYSFUNCTION AND TYPE 2 DIABETES

The association between OSA and metabolic abnormalities such as insulin resistance and type 2 diabetes has been generally characterized using several lines of parallel inquiry.[32,33] These have included correlating metabolic abnormalities to either OSA-related symptoms or OSA severity as assessed by nocturnal recordings of sleep and breathing and assessing whether OSA treatment with positive airway pressure (PAP) therapy has any favorable effects on measured glucose metabolism or glycemic control. Studies on the association between OSA-related symptoms (eg, snoring, witnessed apneas) and glucose metabolism have consistently demonstrated an independent association between OSA and abnormalities such as impaired fasting glucose, glucose intolerance, and type 2 diabetes.[32,33] Consistently, patients with OSA have been shown to have a higher prevalence of type 2 diabetes and metabolic syndrome even after accounting for confounding covariates such as age and BMI. However, the use of surrogate measures to assess OSA (eg, snoring, witnessed apneas) in these studies represents a major weakness, as they provide little insight into the biological mechanisms responsible for the observed association. Fortunately, studies that have used polysomnography to characterize breathing abnormalities during sleep have by and large found an independent association between OSA and metabolic dysfunction.[32,33] OSA severity, as assessed by the AHI and severity of nocturnal oxyhemoglobin desaturation, has been associated with a repertoire of metabolic parameters including higher fasting insulin and glucose levels, a high prevalence of an abnormal oral glucose tolerance test, and impaired insulin sensitivity as assessed by hyperinsulinemic euglycemic clamp.[32,33] Moreover, consideration for confounding factors such as age, BMI, and waist circumference in many of the published studies has provided credence to the hypothesis that OSA is independently, and perhaps causally, associated with metabolic abnormalities including type 2 diabetes.

Given the collective weight of cross-sectional and some longitudinal data linking OSA to insulin resistance, glucose tolerance, and type 2 diabetes, it is surprising that studies on OSA treatment have failed to demonstrate consistent improvements in metabolic function or glycemic control.[32,33] However, much of the available evidence on treatment is based on uncontrolled studies that suffer from a number of methodological flaws including poor adherence to PAP therapy, limited duration of therapy, and small sample size. Thus, definitive conclusions regarding the metabolic implications of OSA therapy with PAP require additional research. Even if well-controlled larger randomized clinical trials in the future demonstrate that PAP therapy does not improve glycemic control, it does not refute the possibility that OSA can induce metabolic abnormalities that can eventually lead to type 2 diabetes. Indeed, several animal and human studies have shown that intermittent hypoxia and sleep fragmentation can initiate a repertoire of pathophysiological effects that can alter normal glucose homeostasis. Exposure to conditions of sustained or intermittent hypoxia can decrease in insulin sensitivity and impair insulin secretion, defects that are fundamental to the pathogenesis of type 2 diabetes. Thus, OSA is likely to be of relevance in the older adult who is likely to have a higher predisposition for OSA and for metabolic dysfunction. Moreover, OSA-related disruption of sleep continuity may also adversely affect glucose metabolism. Although empirical data on the effects of sleep fragmentation are limited, 2 independent groups have demonstrated negative effects of sleep fragmentation on insulin sensitivity in normal subjects.[34,35] The mechanisms through which intermittent hypoxemia and sleep fragmentation could affect glucose metabolism are summarized in **Fig. 2**:

1. Alterations in sympathetic nervous system activity
2. Changes in activity of hypothalamic-pituitary-adrenal (HPA) axis
3. Formation of reactive oxygen species
4. Increases in inflammatory cytokines (ie, interleukin-6) and tumor necrosis factor-α and adipocyte derived factors (ie, leptin, adiponectin, and resistin).[36]

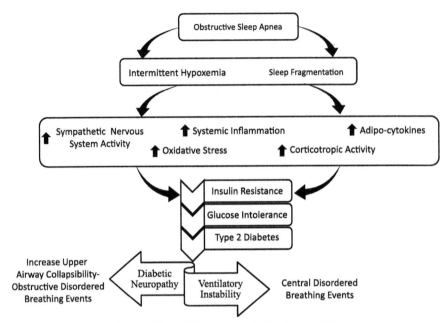

Fig. 2. Associations and causal links OSA and metabolic abnormalities.

TYPE 2 DIABETES AS A RISK FACTOR FOR OBSTRUCTIVE SLEEP APNEA

Although much of the foregoing discussion has focused on OSA as a risk factor for metabolic conditions, the possibility of reverse causation (ie, metabolic conditions such as type 2 diabetes leading to OSA) needs to be also considered (see **Fig. 2**). Indeed, several clinic-based studies have shown that patients with type 2 diabetes are more likely to have IA and central sleep apnea.[37–42] A remarkable feature across these studies is the observation that coexisting autonomic neuropathy substantially increases the prevalence of OSA and central sleep apnea in these patients. Nonetheless, numerous methodological limitations in the available studies prohibit inferences regarding cause and effect and greatly limit the generalizability of the available data. Such issues notwithstanding, investigators from the Sleep Heart Health Study[6] have shown that even after adjusting for confounders such as obesity and prevalent cardiovascular disease, middle-aged and older adults with longstanding type 2 diabetes in the general community are more likely to show evidence of periodic breathing during sleep. Surprisingly, no differences were observed between diabetic and nondiabetic subjects in the frequency of obstructive events. Mechanisms underlying the higher prevalence of central sleep apnea in people with type 2 diabetes are not well understood. Animal models with chemically induced diabetes suggest that abnormal ventilatory responses to hypoxia and/or hypercapnia may be partially responsible. Studies in diabetic patients also show that abnormalities in O_2 ad CO_2 sensitivity may have an important role in increasing respiratory control instability during sleep.[43,44] Whether diabetes also contributes to mechanical alterations in the upper airway and thus increases upper airway collapsibility during sleep remains an open question.

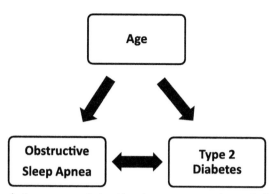

Fig. 3. Interactions between age, obstructive sleep apnea, and type 2 diabetes.

INTERACTIONS OF AGE, SLEEP APNEA, AND TYPE 2 DIABETES

It is also possible that age itself may interact with OSA and augment the predisposition for type 2 diabetes (**Fig. 3**). Although the exact mechanisms for the age-related susceptibility to type 2 diabetes are not known, glucose-stimulated insulin sensitivity and insulin secretion decline with age and result in fasting and postprandial hyperglycemia.[45] In older adults, OSA may accelerate the age-related progression to glucose intolerance and eventually to type 2 diabetes because of the OSA-induced increase in sympathetic nervous system activation and oxidative stress, which, in turn, can decrease peripheral insulin sensitivity and secretion. Conversely, it is also possible that that type 2 diabetes may augment the known effects of age-related risk of OSA. Decreases in muscle function with older age may be hastened in the presence of type 2 diabetes. Insulin resistance and dysglycemia are known risk factors for accelerated muscle loss that results because of decreased stimulation of protein synthesis pathways and increased activation of protein degradation pathways.[31] Thus, age and type 2 diabetes may heighten each other's impact on upper airway function and amplify the risk of OSA. Whether these interactions between age, sleep apnea, and type 2 diabetes exist and whether they are either additive or multiplicative remain to be determined. Such limitations notwithstanding, there is little doubt that the past decade has seen major advances in the understanding of the associations between sleep apnea, glucose intolerance, insulin resistance, and type 2 diabetes. Despite the remarkable advancements, the enthusiasm to implicate causal bidirectional links between OSA and type 2 diabetes has to be somewhat tempered by the fact that both conditions share common risk factors such as obesity. Thus, the challenge that lies ahead is the need to collect additional evidence that will support the hypothesis of a causal association and help define whether age modifies these associations, particularly given that both conditions are common in older adults. A multidisciplinary effort with expertise from various specialties in medicine will provide the foundation on which the complex tapestry that connects age, sleep apnea, and type 2 diabetes can be unwound. Fortunately, the interest in the overlap of these conditions is in its infancy, and a substantial work lies ahead to enhance the ability to answer fundamental questions regarding the bidirectional association between OSA and type 2 diabetes.

REFERENCES

1. US Department of Health and Human Services. Wake up America: a national sleep alert. Bethesda (MD): The Commission; 1993.

2. Vaessen TJ, Overeem S, Sitskoorn MM. Cognitive complaints in obstructive sleep apnea. Sleep Med Rev 2014. [Epub ahead of print].

3. Konecny T, Kara T, Somers VK. Obstructive sleep apnea and hypertension: an update. Hypertension 2014;63(2):203–9.

4. Kasai T, Floras JS, Bradley TD. Sleep apnea and cardiovascular disease: a bidirectional relationship. Circulation 2012;126(12):1495–510.

5. Iftikhar IH, Khan MF, Das A, et al. Meta-analysis: continuous positive airway pressure improves insulin resistance in patients with sleep apnea without diabetes. Ann Am Thorac Soc 2013;10(2):115–20.

6. Resnick HE, Redline S, Shahar E, et al. Diabetes and sleep disturbances: findings from the Sleep Heart Health Study. Diabetes Care 2003;26(3):702–9.

7. Foster GD, Sanders MH, Millman R, et al. Obstructive sleep apnea among obese patients with type 2 diabetes. Diabetes Care 2009;32(6):1017–9.

8. Punjabi NM. The epidemiology of adult obstructive sleep apnea. Proc Am Thorac Soc 2008;5(2):136–43.

9. Young T, Evans L, Finn L, et al. Estimation of the clinically diagnosed proportion of sleep apnea syndrome in middle-aged men and women. Sleep 1997;20(9):705–6.

10. Ancoli-Israel S. Sleep and aging: prevalence of disturbed sleep and treatment considerations in older adults. J Clin Psychiatry 2005;66(Suppl 9):24–30.

11. Ancoli-Israel S, Kripke DF, Klauber MR, et al. Sleep-disordered breathing in community-dwelling elderly. Sleep 1991;14(6):486–95.

12. Ancoli-Israel S, Kripke DF, Klauber MR, et al. Natural history of sleep disordered breathing in community dwelling elderly. Sleep 1993;16(8 Suppl):S25–9.

13. Bixler EO, Vgontzas AN, Ten HT, et al. Effects of age on sleep apnea in men: I. Prevalence and severity. Am J Respir Crit Care Med 1998;157(1):144–8.

14. Duran J, Esnaola S, Rubio R, et al. Obstructive sleep apnea–hypopnea and related clinical features in a population-based sample of subjects aged 30 to 70 yr. Am J Respir Crit Care Med 2001;163(3 Pt 1):685–9.

15. Mehra R, Stone KL, Blackwell T, et al. Prevalence and correlates of sleep-disordered breathing in older men: osteoporotic fractures in men sleep study. J Am Geriatr Soc 2007;55(9):1356–64.

16. Young T, Shahar E, Nieto FJ, et al. Predictors of sleep-disordered breathing in community-dwelling adults: the Sleep Heart Health Study. Arch Intern Med 2002;162(8):893–900.

17. Ancoli-Israel S, Gehrman P, Kripke DF, et al. Long-term follow-up of sleep disordered breathing in older adults. Sleep Med 2001;2(6):511–6.

18. Sforza E, Gauthier M, Crawford-Achour E, et al. A 3-year longitudinal study of sleep disordered breathing in the elderly. Eur Respir J 2012;40(3):665–72.

19. Newman AB, Nieto FJ, Guidry U, et al. Relation of sleep-disordered breathing to cardiovascular disease risk factors: the Sleep Heart Health Study. Am J Epidemiol 2001;154(1):50–9.

20. Redline S, Kirchner HL, Quan SF, et al. The effects of age, sex, ethnicity, and sleep-disordered breathing on sleep architecture. Arch Intern Med 2004; 164(4):406–18.

21. Bliwise DL. Epidemiology of age-dependence in sleep disordered beathing (SDB) in old age: the Bay Area sleep cohort (BASC). Sleep Med Clin 2009; 4(1):57–64.

22. Bliwise DL, Colrain IM, Swan GE, et al. Incident sleep disordered breathing in old age. J Gerontol A Biol Sci Med Sci 2010;65(9):997–1003.

23. Eikermann M, Jordan AS, Chamberlin NL, et al. The influence of aging on pharyngeal collapsibility during sleep. Chest 2007;131(6):1702–9.

24. Strohl KP, Butler JP, Malhotra A. Mechanical properties of the upper airway. Compr Physiol 2012;2(3):1853–72.
25. Endeshaw Y. Clinical characteristics of obstructive sleep apnea in community-dwelling older adults. J Am Geriatr Soc 2006;54(11):1740–4.
26. American Diabetes Association. Diagnosis and classification of diabetes mellitus. Diabetes Care 2014;37(Suppl 1):S81–90.
27. Chen L, Magliano DJ, Zimmet PZ. The worldwide epidemiology of type 2 diabetes mellitus—present and future perspectives. Nat Rev Endocrinol 2012; 8(4):228–36.
28. Wild S, Roglic G, Green A, et al. Global prevalence of diabetes: estimates for the year 2000 and projections for 2030. Diabetes Care 2004;27(5):1047–53.
29. Adeghate E, Schattner P, Dunn E. An update on the etiology and epidemiology of diabetes mellitus. Ann N Y Acad Sci 2006;1084:1–29.
30. Narayan KM, Boyle JP, Geiss LS, et al. Impact of recent increase in incidence on future diabetes burden: U.S., 2005-2050. Diabetes Care 2006;29(9):2114–6.
31. Kalyani RR, Corriere M, Ferrucci L. Age-related and disease-related muscle loss: the effect of diabetes, obesity, and other diseases. Lancet Diabetes Endocrinol 2014. [Epub ahead of print].
32. Punjabi NM, Ahmed MM, Polotsky VY, et al. Sleep-disordered breathing, glucose intolerance, and insulin resistance. Respir Physiol Neurobiol 2003;136(2–3): 167–78.
33. Punjabi NM. Do sleep disorders and associated treatments impact glucose metabolism? Drugs 2009;69(Suppl 2):13–27.
34. Tasali E, Leproult R, Ehrmann DA, et al. Slow-wave sleep and the risk of type 2 diabetes in humans. Proc Natl Acad Sci U S A 2008;105(3):1044–9.
35. Stamatakis KA, Punjabi NM. Effects of sleep fragmentation on glucose metabolism in normal subjects. Chest 2010;137(1):95–101.
36. Aurora RN, Punjabi NM. Obstructive sleep apnoea and type 2 diabetes mellitus: a bidirectional association. Lancet Respir Med 2013;1(4):329–38.
37. Guilleminault C, Briskin JG, Greenfield MS, et al. The impact of autonomic nervous system dysfunction on breathing during sleep. Sleep 1981;4(3):263–78.
38. Rees PJ, Prior JG, Cochrane GM, et al. Sleep apnoea in diabetic patients with autonomic neuropathy. J R Soc Med 1981;74(3):192–5.
39. Catterall JR, Calverley PM, Ewing DJ, et al. Breathing, sleep, and diabetic autonomic neuropathy. Diabetes 1984;33(11):1025–7.
40. Mondini S, Guilleminault C. Abnormal breathing patterns during sleep in diabetes. Ann Neurol 1985;17(4):391–5.
41. Ficker JH, Dertinger SH, Siegfried W, et al. Obstructive sleep apnoea and diabetes mellitus: the role of cardiovascular autonomic neuropathy. Eur Respir J 1998;11(1): 14–9.
42. Bottini P, Dottorini ML, Cristina CM, et al. Sleep-disordered breathing in nonobese diabetic subjects with autonomic neuropathy. Eur Respir J 2003;22(4):654–60.
43. Nishimura M, Miyamoto K, Suzuki A, et al. Ventilatory and heart rate responses to hypoxia and hypercapnia in patients with diabetes mellitus. Thorax 1989;44(4): 251–7.
44. Weisbrod CJ, Eastwood PR, O'Driscoll G, et al. Abnormal ventilatory responses to hypoxia in type 2 diabetes. Diabet Med 2005;22(5):563–8.
45. Basu R, Breda E, Oberg AL, et al. Mechanisms of the age-associated deterioration in glucose tolerance: contribution of alterations in insulin secretion, action, and clearance. Diabetes 2003;52(7):1738–48.

Index

Note: Page numbers of article titles are in **boldface** type.

Clin Geriatr Med 31 (2015) 149–154
http://dx.doi.org/10.1016/S0749-0690(14)00124-4
0749-0690/15/$ – see front matter © 2015 Elsevier Inc. All rights reserved.

geriatric.theclinics.com

Moving?

Make sure your subscription moves with you!

To notify us of your new address, find your **Clinics Account Number** (located on your mailing label above your name), and contact customer service at:

Email: journalscustomerservice-usa@elsevier.com

800-654-2452 (subscribers in the U.S. & Canada)
314-447-8871 (subscribers outside of the U.S. & Canada)

Fax number: 314-447-8029

Elsevier Health Sciences Division
Subscription Customer Service
3251 Riverport Lane
Maryland Heights, MO 63043

*To ensure uninterrupted delivery of your subscription, please notify us at least 4 weeks in advance of move.